Basic Principles of Radiographic Exposure

Basic Principles of Radiographic Exposure

Dianne C. De Vos
Program Director
School of Radiography
Pascack Valley Hospital
Westwood, New Jersey

Lea & Febiger • Philadelphia • London
1990

Lea & Febiger
600 Washington Square
Philadelphia, PA 19106-4198
U.S.A.
(215) 922-1330

Lea & Febiger (UK) Ltd.
145a Croydon Road
Beckenham, Kent BR3 3RB
U.K.

Library of Congress Cataloging in Publication Data

De Vos, Dianne.
    Principles of radiographic exposure / Dianne De Vos.
        p.   cm.
    Bibliography: p.
    Includes index.
    ISBN 0-8121-1222-9
    1. Radiography, Medical—Exposure.   I. Title.
    [DNLM: 1. Radiography—programmed instruction.   2. Technology,
Radiologic—programmed instruction.   WN 18 D512p]
RC78.D475   1989
616.07'572—dc20
DNLM/DLC
for Library of Congress   89-12281
                                                                     CIP

PRINTED IN THE UNITED STATES OF AMERICA

Print number: 5   4   3   2   1

DEDICATION

To my husband, Johnny
my very best friend

Preface

Radiographic exposure is a complex area of radiography to teach—and to learn. This book is designed to give the student a clear understanding of how to formulate techniques of radiographic exposure. It does so by progressing, in a step-by-step, logical sequence, from discussions of x-ray production and properties of x-rays to x-ray-tube rating and coding charts. Comprehension of each new chapter depends on mastery of the previous one; if a student cannot figure mAs, he or she is unable to use the formulas to figure long- and short-scale contrast.

To reinforce comprehension, most chapters include laboratory experiments that are to be worked out by the student. All chapters contain review questions that serve as a means of self-testing. The answers to these questions are provided at the back of the book. Additional general review questions and answers are also included.

It is my hope that this text will help to make a sometimes difficult subject a little easier to digest. Radiographers who are able to use a radiographic machine well are great assets to the health care facility in which they are employed.

Westwood, New Jersey   DIANNE C. DE VOS

Contents

1

X-Ray Production and Properties of X-Rays

OBJECTIVES *After completion of this chapter with the labs, the student radiographer should be able to:*

1. State simply how x-rays are produced.

2. List and identify the portions of a simple x-ray tube.

3. State why x-rays are useful in medicine.

4. List the four distinct tissue types found in humans with regard to x-ray penetration.

5. List the four basic qualities of a radiograph.

6. List the six main properties of x-rays.

To understand the principles of radiographic exposure, one has to have some idea of how x-rays are produced and for what they are used.

X-rays are a small portion of the electromagnetic spectrum. These radiations are found at the extremely short wavelength portion of the spectrum. At this point, the wavelengths are usually measured in Angstrom units (1 Angstrom unit (1 Å) = 10^{-10} or one ten-billionth meter). The useful range for diagnostic radiography is about 0.1 to 0.5 Angstrom units. The shorter the wavelengths of these x-ray waves or photons, the more penetrating they are.

The x-ray beams that diagnostic radiographers use are produced in x-ray tubes. An x-ray tube is an inefficient piece of equipment (Fig. 1–1). Approximately 99.8% of the energy produced in the tube is converted into heat. Only about 0.2% is actually converted into x-ray photons.

How are these x-rays produced?

1. Electrons must be produced in a stream.
2. This electron stream must be set into rapid motion.
3. The electron stream must be stopped suddenly.

In what type of tube are they produced?

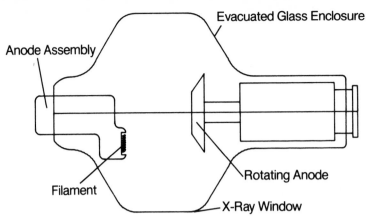

Fig. 1–1. Simple x-ray tube.

1. Evacuated glass envelope.
2. Cathode end or side (electron stream origin).
3. Anode end or side (tungsten target to stop electron stream).

What is the purpose of using x-rays in medicine?

X-rays are extremely penetrating rays. X-rays penetrate all matter according to the density of that matter. Humans are made up of four distinct tissue types in regard to x-ray beams. These tissue types are

1. Bone tissue—most dense or radiopaque.
2. Liquid tissue.
3. Fat or adipose tissue.
4. Air tissue—least dense or radiolucent.

Because of the differences in tissue density, the x-ray beams pass easily through some body areas and have a more difficult time penetrating others. Therefore, the exiting x-ray beam causes different density shadows on the processed radiographic film. A processed radiographic film is a series of shadows of different densities (Fig. 1–2).

All radiographic films demonstrate four basic qualities:

1. Sufficient density (the overall blackening of the film).
2. Proper contrast (differences between extreme blacks and whites on the film).
3. Maximum detail (sharpness of contour lines).
4. Minimum distortion and magnification (all films have magnification because we radiograph three-dimensional (3-D) objects and place them as a two-dimensioned (2-D) image).

The following are the properties of x-rays:

1. Have extremely penetrating electromagnetic waves (this is the reason for the profession of radiography).

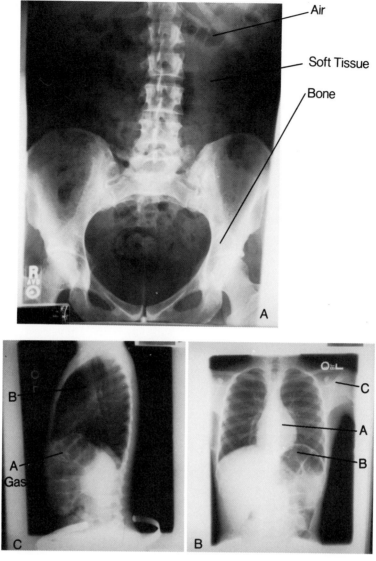

Fig. 1–2. Radiographs that demonstrate different tissue densities of the body. **A.** Abdomen: anterior posterior projection. **B.** Chest: posterior-anterior projection; a. heart; b. gas or air under left lung; c. bone tissue. **C.** Chest: lateral projection; a. gas or air under left lung; b. lung tissue.

2. Produce scattered and secondary radiation (this is why you must learn the principles of radiographic exposure).
3. Cause fluorescence of certain crystals (fluoroscopy and intensifying screens).
4. Cause biologic changes (this is why you must learn radiation protection and radiation biology).
5. Are heterogeneous, or have many different wavelengths (this is why you must learn about filtration).

6. Affect photographic or radiographic film (this is why you must study film processing).
7. Travel in straight lines.
8. Travel at the speed of light.
9. Cannot be focused by a lens.
10. Are electrically neutral.
11. Diverge from the source.

1. X-rays consist of only a small portion of the _____ spectrum.

2. X-rays consist of extremely _____ wavelengths.
   a. Long   b. Short   c. Equal

3. X-rays are measured in _____ units.

4. The useful range of diagnostic radiography is about _____ to _____. (answer to question 3)

5. The shorter the wavelength, the more _____ the x-ray photon.

6. Most energy produced in an x-ray tube is converted into _____.

7. List the three conditions necessary to produce x-rays in a tube.

8. List the three main portions of a simple x-ray tube.

9. List the four tissue types of the body.

10. All radiographic films demonstrate four basic qualities. State them.

11. List the properties of x-rays.

LABS

LAB No. 1

Necessary Equipment

1. Energized x-ray room
2. Cassette with film (10 × 12 or 14 × 17 inches)
3. X-ray phantom (skull or abdomen)
4. Film processor

Take a radiograph of any x-ray phantom. Use a collimated beam that is smaller than the film size.

Observe the radiograph to see the following properties of x-rays:

1. Extremely penetrating. The radiographic image does not look like the phantom.
2. Produce scattered and secondary radiation. Notice the film blackening outside collimator lines.
3. Affect radiographic film. There is an image on the film.

4. Cannot be focused. The beam passed through the collimator mirrors.
5. Diverge from the source. This can be observed by changing the focal film distance.

LAB No. 2

Necessary Equipment

1. Energized x-ray room
2. Empty hinged cassette

Open an empty cassette. Place it on the radiographic table. Darken the room. Expose the intensifying screens. While exposure is in progress, observe through the lead glass window. You can observe that x-rays cause certain crystals to fluoresce.

▬ *2*

Four Prime Factors of Radiographic Exposure

OBJECTIVES *After completion of this chapter with the labs, the student radiographer should be able to:*

1. List the four prime factors of a radiographic exposure.

2. Convert amperes to milliamperage.

3. Convert seconds to milliseconds.

4. Figure problems using milliamperage and time of exposure.

5. Alter milliamperage or time to obtain given mAs values.

6. Discuss kilovoltage as it pertains to penetration or quality of the x-ray beam.

7. Figure problems to determine minimum kVp levels for patients.

8. Use a caliper stick.

9. Demonstrate how the x-rays diverge from their source.

10. State the commonly used focal-film distances used in a radiology department.

Many factors come into play when producing a radiographic film. We will deal with the prime factors in this chapter. They are

1. Milliamperage (mA).
2. Time of exposure, measured in seconds (s) or milliseconds (ms).
3. Kilovoltage (kVp).
4. Distance—focal-film distance (FFD).

MILLIAMPERAGE

X-ray tube currents are measured in milliamperes. One milliampere is equal to 1/1000 of an ampere. An ampere is a measurement of electric current. Commonly, x-ray machines use milliamperes that range from about 25 to about 1500.

The time of the x-ray exposure is governed by a timer. Times of x-ray exposures can be as short as 0.001 second (1 ms) or as long as about 8 seconds. This is the reason that both milliseconds and seconds are used relative to times of exposure. The term milli means 1000. Therefore, 1 millisecond equals 1/1000 of a second. There are 1000 milliseconds in 1 second.

Tube current (mA) along with the exposure time (s) equals mAs.

$$mA \times s = mAs$$

mA and time are inversely proportional. It is a good idea to try to talk and think in terms of mAs rather than mA and time. If a machine has settings of 300 mA and 1/10 second, for example, you should try to think of it as 30 mAs rather than 300 mA and 1/10 second.

$$300 \ (mA) \times 1/10 \ (s) = 30 \ mAs$$

$$\frac{300}{1} \times 1/10 = \frac{300}{10} = 30$$

$$300 \times 0.1 = 30$$

When the machine setting for time is measured in milliseconds (ms), you must convert the milliseconds to seconds before figuring the mAs. If the machine has settings of 300 mA and 100 ms, the first thing to do is to convert the milliseconds into seconds.

$$\frac{100}{1000} = 1/10$$

Divide the ms by 1000. $1000\overline{)100.0}^{\ 0.1}$

Now multiply the mA × s. 300 × 0.1 = 30

If you forget to change the milliseconds to seconds, the answer will be wrong. No matter what the settings are, mA × s is always the mAs.

$$100 \times 1/10 = 10$$

$$200 \times 1/20 = 10$$

$$300 \times 1/30 = 10$$

The mAs is exactly the same for each of the above.

The mAs is considered the *amount* or *quantity* of x-radiation we are using to get the x-ray exposure. If for some reason a mistake is made in selecting the mA or time factor, the amount will not be what is needed:

$$100 \times 1/10 = 10$$

$$100 \times 1/20 = 5$$

If you need 10 mAs but only have 5, the finished radiograph will have one-half the density that is needed.

You can obtain the mAs with a particular mA and time. Let us say that we must use 10 mAs for a particular radiographic examination. The patient has a problem and cannot hold still for 1/10 of a second. What can be done about this?

Suppose the machine has an mA station of 500. You know that if you use the 500 mA station, you can use less time than if you use the 100 mA station. But what time should be used?

$$mA \times s = mAs$$

One side of the equation must equal the other side.

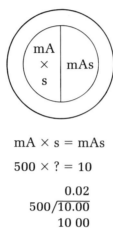

$$mA \times s = mAs$$

$$500 \times ? = 10$$

$$\begin{array}{r} 0.02 \\ 500\overline{)10.00} \\ 10\ 00 \end{array}$$

The time to use with a 500 mA station is 0.02 s or 1/50 s or 20 ms. Let us work this another way. Suppose you decide that the exposure time to be used for the same patient should be no more than 1/40 (0.025). What mA station should you use?

$$mA \times s \quad = mAs$$

$$? \times 0.025 = 10$$

$$\begin{array}{r} 400. \\ 0.025\overline{)10.000.} \\ 123 \qquad 123 \end{array}$$

Now you can see that you can solve for any one unknown factor if you know the other two. It is also easy to check your answer. **Always remember:** mA × s = mAs.

$$0.02 \times 500 = 10$$

$$0.025 \times 400 = 10$$

I am sure that at some time you will work with machines that do not have separate mA and time stations. Some of the newer machines and many portable machines are equipped only with mAs settings. These machines are easy to use, but the radiographer has no control over the time setting. This usually is not a problem. If, however, you need or want a long exposure time, it cannot be accomplished.

KILOVOLTAGE (kVp)

X-ray voltage is measured in peak kilovolts (kVp). Each kilovolt is equal to 1000 volts of electric potential. The term kilo means 1000. You can see that x-ray machines operate with high voltages.

Most diagnostic x-ray machines operate at kVp levels of between 40 and 150. As the kVp increases, the x-ray wavelengths become shorter and more penetrating. The kVp is the penetrating power of the x-ray machine. This is referred to as the *quality* of the x-ray beam, the strength of the beam. With most x-ray machines, the radiographer is able to adjust the kVp setting by 1 or 2 kVp. It usually is an easier adjustment than changing the mAs.

Because kVp is the penetrating power of the x-ray beam, at some point we must figure the necessary kVp to be used with an object. You must have enough penetration to get the x-ray beam through the object to carry the information to the film.

This should be accomplished with the use of a caliper stick. This is a device used to measure anatomic thickness in centimeters. Before students are able to figure radiographic technique, they must be instructed on the proper use of a caliper stick. The antomic measurement is the distance the x-ray beam travels through the patient. It does not include the space between the patient and the film.

The rule of thumb for figuring **minimum kVp** is:

$$2 \times \text{cm thickness} + 25 \text{ for three-phase equipment}$$

$$2 \times \text{cm thickness} + 30 \text{ for single-phase equipment}$$

As an example, you measure a knee to be radiographed. The knee measures 14 cm (Fig. 2–1).

Three-phase equipment: $14 \times 2 + 25$
$28 + 25 = 53$ is minimum kVp

Single-phase equipment: $14 \times 2 = 28$
$28 + 30 = 58$ is minimum kVp

(This rule does not pertain to chest radiographs, because the chest is so much less dense than the rest of the body. Chest radiographs should be taken using high kVp.)

The kVp usually can be increased from the minimum kVp, but it can not be reduced, because the object will absorb too much of a weak, nonpenetrating x-ray beam.

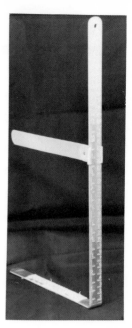

Fig. 2–1. Caliper stick to obtain the proper measurement (in centimeters) of patients.

FOCAL-FILM DISTANCE

X-rays follow the inverse square law, which means two things:

1. The x-ray beam diverges from the source or focal spot. The beam becomes larger on all four sides as the distance increases.
2. As this beam becomes larger or more spread out, it becomes weaker.

If the beam is weaker, it will affect the density (overall blackening) of the radiograph film. For this reason, you must be able to figure how much more or less mAs is needed when a change in the focal-film distance (FFD) is necessary.

Radiology departments use a variety of FFD. The most common distances are 40 and 72 inches. The FFD play a part in the magnification of the radiographic image. This is explained fully in Chapter 5.

1. List the four prime factors of a radiographic exposure.

2. X-ray tube currents are measured in _____.

3. The usual range of x-ray exposure times is _____ to _____.

4. How are x-ray exposure times measured? (Two ways)

5. What does the term milli mean?

6. mA and time are _____ proportional to each other.

7. Figure the mAs for the following:
   - a. 300 mA   1/20 s
   - b. 400 mA   0.02 s
   - c. 200 mA   25 ms

8. Figure the time for the following:
   - a. 300 mA   45 mAs   ? s   ? ms
   - b. 400 mA   20 mAs   ? s   ? ms
   - c. 600 mA   5 mAs   ? s   ? ms

9. Figure the mA station for the following:
   - a. 30 mAs   1/60 s
   - b. 40 mAs   0.1 s
   - c. 6 mAs   50 ms

10. One kVp is equal to _____ volts.

11. As kVp is increased, the wavelengths become _____.
    - a. Longer
    - b. Shorter
    - c. Wider

12. The kVp is the _____ of the x-ray exposure.
    1. Quantity   2. Quality   3. Amount   4. Penetrating power
    a. All of the above   b. 1 and 2   c. 2 and 3   d. 2 and 4

13. What is the rule of thumb to determine minimum kVp?

14. Why is it possible to use kVp that is higher than the minimum but not kvP that is lower than the minimum?

15. As the x-ray beam diverges from the source it becomes _____.
    - a. Weaker
    - b. Stronger

LAB No. 1

Necessary Equipment

1. X-ray step wedge (penetrometer)
2. 10 × 12-inch cassette with film
3. Energized x-ray room
4. Film processor
5. Two sheets of lead rubber shields

Figure a radiographic technique for 10 mAs by using four different mA and time stations, i.e., 100 × 1/10, 200 × 1/20, 300 × 1/30, and 400 × 1/40.

Take four separate exposures on the 10 × 12-inch cassette. Use the same kVp, FFD, and collimation. Make sure you use the lead rubber to shield the cassette portion not used for each exposure. Process the film and observe that each exposure gives the same radiographic film density.

You should be able to observe that no matter how you arrive at the mAs, mA × s = mAs.

If you notice that all the films do not have equal density, the x-ray machine should be callibrated.

LAB No. 2

Necessary Equipment

1. Skull phantom (not skeleton skull)
2. 10 × 12-inch cassette with film (2)
3. Energized x-ray room
4. Processor
5. Caliper stick

Measure the skull phantom for minimum kVp (see pg. 10). Expose one film by using this minimum kVp and the other by using 10 kVp less. (Ask your instructor for additional parts of the technique mA and time.) Process the films and observe that the radiograph with less than minimum kVp even with more mAs is not sufficiently penetrated by the x-ray beam.

LAB No. 3

Necessary Equipment

1. Energized x-ray room
2. Processor
3. 10 × 12-inch cassettes with film (3)
4. Rad check exposure device or pocket dosimeter

Place one cassette under the collimator set at 50 inches from the film. Place the dosimeter or rad check in the center of the cassette. Collimate the field to 9 × 9 inches. Expose this film; use 10 mAs, 60 kVp. Record the millirad (mrad). Develop the film. Repeat with the second cassette. Move the distance to 40 inches. Do not change the collimation. Reset the rad check or dosimeter and place it in the center of the film. Expose using the same mAs and kVp. Record the millirad; develop film no. 2. Repeat with the third cassette. Move the FFD to 30 inches. Do not change the collimation. Reset the rad check or dosimeter and place it in the center of the film. Expose again using the same mAs and kVp. Record the millirad for the third film and develop the film.

Observe the millirad readings and also the films. You should observe the following:

Film no. 1 will have the least density and the largest image.
Film no. 2 will have more density than film no. 1 with a smaller image.
Film no. 3 will have the most density and the smallest image.

The millirad readings you observed should be the highest for film no. 3 and the lowest for film no. 1.

This lab should prove that as the FFD increases, the density and intensity decreases and vice versa. This lab will also demonstrate the divergence of the x-ray beam.

━ *3*

Radiographic Contrast

OBJECTIVES *After completion of this chapter with the labs, the student radiographer should be able to:*

1. Define radiographic contrast.

2. Differentiate between long and short scale radiographic contrasts.

3. Figure radiographic exposure techniques for lengthening or shortening a radiographic contrast.

4. Defend the use of long scale contrast.

The definition of radiographic contrast is the extreme differences between the blacks and whites of a radiographic image. A radiographic image is a series of shadows of different densities. This is where a good radiographer comes in. We, as technologists, have the ability to change or alter the radiographic contrast.

When we think of contrast, it is usually of two types:

1. Long scale (low scale): many subtle shades of grey.
2. Short scale (high scale): black and white.

Think now of what kVp does. It is the penetrating power of the x-ray beam; therefore, the higher the kVp, the more remnant radiation reaches the radiographic film. In addition, more scattered and secondary radiation reaches the film. When this film is developed, it appears more gray. There are many subtle shades. When you look at a radiograph with this long scale contrast it may appear flat or dull. On closer inspection, however, you can see many small structures that might otherwise blend in with surrounding anatomy. For this reason, most radiologists prefer films that demonstrate long or low scale contrast.

On the other hand, if you use kVp ranges that are low or close to minimum (remember the rule of thumb for determining minimum kVp), the radiographs look relatively black and white. At first glance, they appear more pleasing to the eye. On closer inspection, you should see that the areas in question are usually too dark or too light, i.e., the bony area is clear and less dense tissue is black. If a patient has a small bone tumor, it may not be well demonstrated (it is not penetrated enough), and if an area in question coincides with the dark portions of the film, the radiologist may not be able to visualize this portion adequately.

Another good reason to try to use longer scale contrast in radiography is that the patient receives less radiation when we use low mAs and high kVp. This is an important consideration. In most instances, we are able to either lengthen or shorten the scale of contrast.

Formula to Lengthen the Scale of Contrast (Low Contrast)

To lengthen the scale, you increase the kVp by 15% and decrease the mAs by 50%.

Original technique: 80 kVp
                    20 mAs

1. Increase 80 kVp to 92 kVp. 15% of 80 = 12. 80 + 12 = 92. New kVp. = 92
2. Decrease mAs by 50%. 1/2 of 20 = 10. New mAs = 10. The 80 kVp at 20 mAs will produce equal density as 92 kVp at 10 mAs.

The difference between these two films is that the one with the original technique will be of shorter scale contrast (more black and white), whereas the one with increased kVp and decreased mAs will have a longer scale of contrast (more grays).

Formula to Shorten the Scale of Contrast (High Contrast)

To shorten the scale, you decrease the kVp by 15% and increase the mAs by 2 times.

Original technique: 94 kVp
                    15 mAs

1. Decrease 94 kVp to 80 kVp. 15% of 94 = 14.1. 94 − 14 = 80. New kVp = 80
2. Increase mAs by 2×. 2 × 15 = 30. New mAs = 30. The 94 kVp at 15 mAs will produce equal density as 80 kVp at 30 mAs. Now you can see that it is possible to lengthen or shorten contrast to improve the radiographs.

Now to backtrack and work some mAs, kVp problems:

PROBLEM 1: Original technique: 200 mAs
                              1/10 s
                              66 kVp
                              200 × 1/10 = 20 mAs

Use equal density and longer contrast scale.
New technique: Use 1/2 of 20 mAs. New mAs = 10
              Increase 66 kVp by 15% (10). New kVp = 76

PROBLEM 2: Original technique: 400 mA
                           0.02 s
                           72 kVp

Shorten the scale of contrast and use the 200 mA station.
New technique: 15% of 72 = 10.8 (11). 72 − 11 = 61. New kVp = 61
        Original mA = 8. 400 × 0.02 = 8. New mAs = 16
        16 ÷ 200 = 0.08 s
(**Remember:** to always find original mAs.)

PROBLEM 3: Original technique: 300 mA
                           25 ms
                           88 kVp

Lengthen the scale of contrast and use 1/40 s in time.
New technique: 15% of 88 = 13.2 (13). New kVp = 101
        Original mAs = 7.5. 300 × 0.025 = 7.5. New mAs = 3.75
        (7.5 ÷ 2 = 3.75)
        3.75 ÷ 1/40s = 150 mA
You can easily see that to work problems to shorten or lengthen the scale of contrast, it is important to be able to work the previous problems dealing with mA and time relationship.

Other factors enter into radiographic contrast, and these are discussed in later chapters. These factors include:

1. Film/screen systems.
2. Grids.
3. Subject or patient contrast.
4. Filters.
5. Cones, diaphragms, and collimators.

1. What is the definition of radiographic contrast?

2. Define long or low scale contrast.

3. Define short or high scale contrast.

4. Which type of radiographic contrast usually produces more scattered and secondary radiation? Why?

5. Generally speaking, a radiographer should try to use techniques that utilize:
   a. High kVp − low mAs
   b. High kVp − high mAs
   c. Low kVp − low MaS
   d. Low kVp − high mAs

6. Using the 15% kVp rule for contrast, lengthen the scale of contrast for the following:

Original Technique	New Technique
a. 100 mA	? mAs
1/5 s	? kVp
88 kVp	
b. 200 mA	400 mA
0.05 s	? s
77 kVp	? kVp
c. 300 mA	200 mA
25 ms	? ms
80 kVp	? kVp
d. 200 mA	? mA
1/10 s	0.05 s
90 kVp	? kVp

7. Using the 15% kVp rule for contrast, shorten the scale of contrast for the following:

Original Technique	New Technique
a. 100 mA	? mAs
1/5 s	? kVp
88 kVp	
b. 300 mA	300 mA
0.003 s	? s
94 kVp	? kVp
c. 500 mA	1000 mA
50 ms	? ms
79 kVp	? mVp
d. 400 mA	? mA
1/20 s	25 ms
80 kVp	? kVp

Necessary Equipment

1. Energized x-ray room
2. X-ray step wedge (penetrometer)
3. Processor
4. 10 × 12-inch, cassette filled (2)
5. Lead rubber film blockers

First, expose the step wedge to a technique using 55 kVp and 20 mAs. If this is a good radiographic technique to use in your department, you can continue. If not, get a good short scale contrast technique from your instructor. Try to use kVp in the fifties. After you have obtained your baseline short-scale contrast technique, figure four or five longer scale contrast techniques.

	mAs	kVp
Film No. 1 baseline	20	55
Film No. 2 1 step longer	10	63
Film No. 3 1 step longer than no. 2	5	72
Film No. 4 1 step longer than no. 3	2.5	83
Film No. 5 1 step longer than no. 4	1.25	95
Film No. 6 1 step longer than no. 5	0.66	109

Expose these films using the previous techniques as accurately as possible. Do not change the FFD or collimation. After processing these films, line them up on a viewbox and compare them. Look at the differences between the black and white scales and the gray scales. You can take this lab a step further by using the rad check or dosimeter and exposing it to each of the techniques. Remember to record each millirad reading and reset the device for each exposure. You should observe that the longer the scale of contrast, the less radiation the patient would receive. Also note that you are able to see more information on the longer scale films.

4

Inverse Square Law

As stated in Chapter 2, x-rays diverge from their source or origin. Therefore, the field covered by any given x-ray beam increases as it is moved further from the radiographic film that will contain the radiographic image. The problem is not that the actual field size will enlarge, but that as this x-ray beam is increasing in area, it is decreasing in strength (Fig. 4–1). With this fact in mind, we must be able to calculate what changes in the strength of the beam are necessary to keep the radiographic film density equal.

You have probably already discussed how the inverse square law applies to radiation protection. You know that distance is your best radiation protection device.

The inverse square law states the following:

$$\frac{\text{Intensity 1}}{\text{Intensity 2}} = \frac{\text{Distance 2}^2}{\text{Distance 1}^2}$$

To apply this law:

1. $\dfrac{\text{Intensity (22 mrad)}}{\text{Intensity ?}} = \dfrac{\text{Distance 24 inches}}{\text{Distance 12 inches}}$

2. $\dfrac{22}{?} = \dfrac{24^2}{12^2}$

3. $\dfrac{22}{?} = \dfrac{576}{144}$

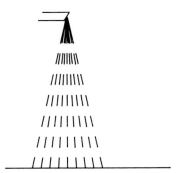

Fig. 4–1. As the x-ray photons diverge, they become weaker because they cover a larger area.

4. Cross-multiply 22 × 144 = 3168
5. 3168 ÷ 576 = 5.5

This calculation means that if you stand 12 inches from an x-radiation source, you receive 22 millirad (mrad). When you move back to 24 inches, you receive only 5.5 millirad of radiation. You can see that the closer you stand to an x-radiation source, the more x-radiation you receive.

This formula changes somewhat when dealing with mAs changes that are necessary if the focal-film distance (FFD) is changed. We make these changes because we want the radiographic images to have the same density.

LONG METHOD

The mAs—distance change formula is as follows:

$$\frac{\text{Old mAs}}{\text{New mAs}} = \frac{\text{Old FFD}^2}{\text{New FFD}^2}$$

Let us apply a technique to the formula.

1. $\dfrac{25}{\quad} = \dfrac{40^2}{60^2}$

2. $\dfrac{25}{\quad} = \dfrac{1600}{3600}$

3. Cross-multiply 25 × 3600 and ÷ 1600 = 56.2

The new mAs is 56.2 to be used with an FFD of 60 inches. Use 56 mAs instead of 25 mAs.

A patient comes to the Radiology Department for an examination of the elbow. The following is the suggested radiographic technique:

100 mA
0.015 s
56 kVp
40-inch FFD

For some reason, you are instructed to use an FFD of 50 inches. Let us put the formula to work:

1. $\dfrac{\text{Old mAs } 100 \times 0.015 = 1.5}{\text{New mAs ?}} = \dfrac{\text{Old FFD } 40}{\text{New FFD } 50}$

2. $\dfrac{1.5}{?} = \dfrac{40^2}{50^2}$

3. $\dfrac{1.5}{?} = \dfrac{1600}{2500}$

4. Cross-multiply $1.5 \times 2500 = 3750$

5. $3750 \div 1600 = 2.34$

Use 2.34 mAs at the 50-inch FFD and the density will be equal to 1.5 at 40-inch FFD

SHORT METHOD

An easier way to figure this formula does not involve the use of such large numbers. To figure the new mAs, simply divide the old FFD into the new FFD. Square this result and multiply by the old mAs.

1.
$$
\begin{array}{r}
1.25 \\
40\overline{)50.00} \\
\underline{40} \\
100 \\
\underline{80} \\
200 \\
\underline{200} \\
\end{array}
$$

2. $1.25 \times 1.25 = 1.56$

3. $1.56 \times 1.5 = 2.34$

You might find this a less cumbersome method to use. Make sure that you figure the mAs before you begin.

Now work a problem with two changes.

Original technique: 200 mA
1/10 s
80 kVp
40-inch FFD

The new technique calls for a longer scale of contrast using a 48-inch FFD.

1. Figure mAs. $200 \times 1/10 = 20$
2. Increase 80 kVp to 92. $80 \times 15\% = 12$. $80 + 12 = 92$
3. When the kVp is changed to 92, the mAs must become 10 instead of 20
4. We now have 10 mAs at 92 kVp. This is to be used with a 40-inch FFD
5. When changing the FFD to 48, the new mAs becomes 14.4 (work inverse square law)

6. The new technique to be used with these changes is: 48-inch FFD, 92 kVp, 14.4 mAs (you probably have to use 15 mAs).

This technique offers the same density with a longer (more gray) scale of contrast.
 Try this one.
Original technique: 300 mA
                    0.05 s
                    100 kVp
                    40-inch FFD
The new technique calls for a shorter scale of contrast with a 46-inch FFD and you must use the 400 mA station.

1. Figure mAs. 300 × 0.05 = 15 mAs
2. Decrease 100 kVp to 85. 100 × 15% = 15. 100 − 15 = 85
3. When kVp is changed to 85, the mAs must become 30 instead of 15
4. We now have 30 mAs at 85 kVp to be used with a 40-inch FFD
5. When changing the FFD to 46 inches, the new mAs becomes 39.6 (40) (use inverse square law formula)
6. When using 40 mAs, if the 400 mA station is used, the new time will be 1/10 (40 ÷ 400 = 0.1 or 1/10. 400 × 1/10 = 40)
7. The new technique to be used with these changes is:
      400 mA
      1/10 s
      85 kVp
      46-inch FFD

This technique offers the same density with a shorter (more black and white) scale of contrast.

1. As x-ray beams diverge from a source they:
   1. Become stronger
   2. Become wider on both sides
   3. Become weaker
   4. Become smaller on both sides
   - a. 1 and 2
   - b. 2 and 3
   - c. 3 and 4
   - d. 1 and 4

2. What is the formula for intensity inverse square law?

3. What is the formula for the mAs-FFD (focal-film distance) relationship?

4. If a radiographer receives 14 millirad of x-radiation at a distance of 4 feet, what is the dose to that radiographer if he moves back to 7 feet?

5. What radiographic technique should be used for the following to keep the radiographic density equal?

Original Technique	New Technique
a. 25 mAs	? mAs
40-inch FFD	45-inch FFD
b. 400 mA	200 mA
1/10 s	? s
60-inch FFD	30-inch FFD
c. 300 mA	300 mA
0.05 s	? s
45-inch FFD	35-inch FFD
d. 300 mA	600 mA
1/10 s	? ms
40-inch FFD	48-inch FFD
80 kVp	92 kVp
e. 400 mA	200 mA
30 ms	? ms
72-inch FFD	40-inch FFD
75 kVp	86 kVp

6. Change the following radiographic technique to one with equal density and a longer scale of contrast.

25 mAs	? mAs
40-inch FFD	25-inch FFD
66 kVp	? kVp

7. Change the following radiographic technique to one with equal density and a shorter scale of contrast.

200 mA	400 mA
50 ms	? ms
99 kVp	? kVp
40-inch FFD	55-inch FFD

8. Which of the following radiographic techniques will offer the most density?

a. 200 mA	b. 300 mA	c. 600 mA
1/10 s	1/30 s	1/60 s
75 kVp	80 kVp	92 kVp

9. Which of the following radiographic techniques will offer the least density?

a. 400 mA	b. 800 mA	c. 200 mA
50 ms	1/40 s	1/10 s
88 kVp	100 kVp	75 kVp

LAB

Necessary Equipment

1. Energized x-ray room (tube that is able to move from 25 to 50 inches)
2. Processor
3. Skull phantom (or any x-ray phantom or wedge step)
4. 9.5 × 9.5-inch cassettes filled (5)

Using a base radiographic lateral skull technique at a 40-inch FFD (10 mAs; 62 kVp),* figure a new radiographic technique for the following new FFD:

a. 50 inches	15.6
b. 45 inches	12.5
c. 30 inches	5.6
d. 25 inches	3.8

If you cannot use the new techniques because of the mA and time stations, try a different base radiographic technique. Use techniques that are as close as possible. Make a note if you use something close but a little different, i.e., you need 15.6 mAs but are able to use 15 mAs. Expose the films and process them. When you change the FFD, try to keep the collimation as close to the original as possible. Compare the films. They should all have the same density. You should note as an additional finding that the films with the short FFD do not have as much detail as those taken with the longer FFD (this is explained in Chapter 5). You can also use the rad check or dosimeter to check each exposure. They should be equal.

---

*This technique works well with a 400 film/screen combination. Check with your clinical instructor regarding a proper radiographic technique.

─ 5

Radiographic Unsharpness

OBJECTIVES *After completion of this chapter with the labs, the student radiographer should be able to:*

1. List the various types of radiographic unsharpness.

2. Explain how to reduce motion unsharpness.

3. List the factors that produce geometric unsharpness. Figure ways to reduce geometric unsharpness.

4. Discuss ways to reduce parallax effect.

5. Work problems to figure either image or object size.

6. Figure the magnification factor of radiographs.

7. Figure the magnification percentage or radiographs.

8. Discuss how true distortion is of influence in radiography. List anatomic areas for which true distortion is used to advantage.

All radiographic films have a certain amount of distortion. For all general purposes, we are radiographing a three-dimensional object and putting the image on a two-dimensional sheet of radiographic film. Therefore, all films have distortion of the object shape. If you radiograph a ball-shaped object, the image will be that of a circle.

Radiographic unsharpness takes several forms, defined as the following:

1. Motion unsharpness.
2. Geometric unsharpness.
3. Inherent unsharpness.
4. Magnification unsharpness (size distortion).
5. Shape distortion.

MOTION UNSHARPNESS

The first, and also the worst, unsharpness is motion. In most instances, a radiographic film that has evidence of motion (patient was moving or breathing) will have to be repeated. Not a good thing to do. The patient receives more x-radiation than is necessary and it is a waste of film and time. There is only one effective way to eliminate motion from films: employ a short exposure time. Radiology departments have a vast array of immobilizing devices that just do not work well. It is virtually impossible to tell a 6-month-old child to hold his breath or to stop moving. When radiographing young children or any uncooperative patient, it is most important to immobilize that individual and also to use a short exposure time. This task is easy if your x-ray machine has high mA stations.

$$100 \text{ mA, } 0.5 \text{ s} = 50 \text{ mAs}$$

$$1000 \text{ mA, } 0.05 \text{ s} = 50 \text{ mAs}$$

It is easy to see that there would be less motion when using an exposure time of 0.05 s instead of 0.5 s. The second exposure time is 10 times faster than the first and the mAs is equal.

If a particular x-ray machine does not have high mA capabilities, you could add 15% to the kVp and cut the exposure time by one half.

$$100 \text{ mA, } 0.5 \text{ s, } 70 \text{ kVp}$$

$$100 \text{ mA, } 0.25 \text{ s, } 81 \text{ kVp}$$

Both exposures offer equal density. The second exposure has a longer scale of contrast. You could carry that another step if you wish:

$$100 \text{ mA, } 0.125 \text{ s, } 93 \text{ kVp}$$

Again, equal density as the previous example. The contrast will be longer. (Do you begin to see the difference between a good radiographer and a "button pusher"?)

GEOMETRIC UNSHARPNESS

The next type of unsharpness deals with geometry. This unsharpness occurs because x-rays are generated on an area (focal spot), and once generated, these x-rays diverge from that source. The x-ray beam cannot begin at infinity; it must begin in some area. X-ray tubes are usually sold with two focal spot sizes (FSS) (Fig. 5–1). These focal spots are determined by the size of the cathode filament. Focal spot sizes vary anywhere from 0.1 to 2.0 mm.

The larger the FSS, the more unsharpness on the film. When the x-ray beam begins its divergence at a smaller area, the image will have less blur (Fig. 5–2).

Geometric unsharpness also depends on the focal-film distance (FFD), the object-film distance (OFD), and the focal-object distance (FOD). There is a formula to determine the amount of geometric unsharpness. It really does nothing more than let you know which film has the least or most amount of geometric unsharpness. It does not necessarily mean that the film with the least

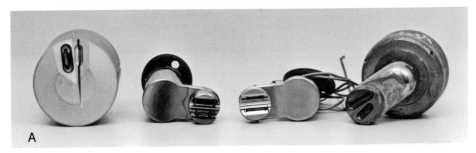

Fig. 5–1. Small and large filaments of a double focus x-ray tube. Notice that the smaller filament is not only shorter but has a smaller diameter and a smaller width.

geometric unsharpness is the best, because another film might have motion or more magnification. It is, however, a good thing to know.

The geometric unsharpness formula states that:

$$\text{Geometric unsharpness} = \frac{\text{Focal spot size (FSS)} \times \text{object-film distance (OFD)}}{\text{Focal-object-distance (FOD)}}$$

Check these numbers: 1.5 is the size of the focal spot, 6 is the OFD, 34 is the FOD. The FFD is 40 inches, because 34 + 6 = 40.

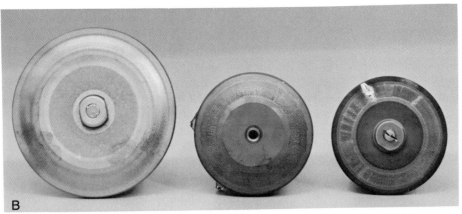

Fig. 5–2. A, Various size focal spots from dismantled x-ray tubes. **B,** Focal spots on anodes.

$$\frac{1.5 \times 6}{34} = 9/34$$

Geometric unsharpness = 9/34 or 0.264

If you could move that object closer to the film, the geometric unsharpness would be less. Suppose you could change the OFD to 4 inches.

$$\frac{1.5 \times 4}{36}$$

$$\frac{1.5 \times 4}{36} = 6/36 = 1/6$$

Geometric unsharpness = 1/6 or 0.166

If you cannot change the OFD (many times it is impossible) and the geometric unsharpness must be reduced, you could increase the FFD:

$$\frac{1.5 \times 6}{44}$$

When the FFD is increased to 50 inches:

$$44 + 6 = 50$$

$$\frac{1.5 \times 6}{44} = 9/44$$

Geometric unsharpness = 9/44 or 0.204

When comparing these figures, you can readily see that it is better to reduce the OFD than to increase the FFD. The FSS can be reduced only within the limits of the tube. Many times the small focal spot cannot be used with high mAs and kVp techniques.

INHERENT UNSHARPNESS

The term inherent means something that is already there or cannot be changed. Inherent unsharpness deals with the film type used and mostly with the type of intensifying screens employed. Whenever intensifying screens are used, the patient receives a smaller dose of x-radiation. In all radiology department radiographers utilize screens for this reason. Most radiographs are produced with the use of intensifying screens. These intensifying screens do cause a limitation of detail. When the x-ray beam strikes the intensifying screen, visible light is given off from that screen's flourescence. This light diverges as it travels to the radiographic film and causes a certain amount of distortion or loss of detail. (Chapter 8 includes a more in-depth discussion of intensifying screens.) The type of radiographic film used also causes a slight bit of unsharpness.
Radiographic film demonstrates one other type of unsharpness called the

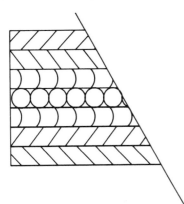

Fig. 5–3. Demonstration of the parallax effect with an angled central ray. The central ray enters and exits at different portions of the radiographic film.

parallax effect. The parallax effect is the distortion caused by the thickness of the film. Radiographic film usually consists of seven layers and has a thickness of between 0.22 and 0.25 mm. This means that the image from one side to the other has a magnification factor. This factor usually is of no consequence to the radiograph. The only time in which it could become a problem is if you are using a short FFD or a large angle of the central ray. The angled central ray will move the top area of the image further from the bottom image (Fig. 5–3).

MAGNIFICATION UNSHARPNESS (SIZE DISTORTION)

As stated previously, all radiographs have some magnification distortion. It is easy to figure the image size by using the following formula:

$$\frac{\text{Object size}}{\text{Image size}} = \frac{\text{Focal-object distance (FOD)}}{\text{Focal-film distance (FFD)}}$$

Consider these numbers:

$$\frac{6}{?} = \frac{36}{40}$$

Cross-multiply 6 × 40 = 240

240 ÷ 36 = 6.66

The image will measure 6.66 inches on the radiographic film. If you want to figure the magnification factor, use the following:

$$\text{Magnification factor} = \frac{\text{Focal-film distance}}{\text{Focal-object distance}}$$

So if:

$$\frac{40}{36} = 1.1$$

The magnification factor is 1.1.

When you want to figure the percent of magnification, use the following:

$$\frac{\text{Object-film distance}}{\text{Target-object distance}} \times 100$$

For example:

$$\frac{4 \times 100}{36}$$

$$\frac{400}{36} = 11.1\%$$

Usually, it is better to be able to figure the magnification factor or the percent of magnification because there is more information. Just to know that the image size is 6.6 inches does not mean as much to you as to know that the magnification is 11.1%. It might be helpful to know the image size if you want to use a particular film size for an examination. For example, you must radiograph a humerus that measures 11 inches in length. You want to use a film that measures 24 × 30 cm. Will this humerus fit lengthwise on this film with an FFD of 40 inches and an OFD of 6 inches?

$$\frac{11}{?} = \frac{34}{40}$$

Cross-multiply 11 × 40 = 440

440 ÷ 34 = 12.9

The image will measure 12.9 inches and the film is 11.81 inches (30 ÷ 2.54 = 11.81 inches). The entire humerus will not fit lengthwise on this film. What is the percent of magnification for the previous example?

$$\frac{6 \times 100}{34}$$

$$\frac{600}{34} = 17.6\%$$

SHAPE DISTORTION

You know by now that all films demonstrate some size distortion. They also demonstrate shape distortion. Sometimes we use this distortion to our advantage in positioning the patient or with angling the central ray. Think of what

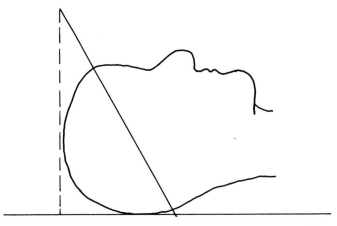

Fig. 5–4. True distortion angling of central ray to remove superimposition of the bones of the skull.

happens to the image on an apical lordotic chest radiograph. The central ray is angled about 15° cephalad (toward the head) to "move" the clavicles out of the area of the apex of the lungs. As you progress through your course, you will find many instances in which you must angle the central ray or the patient to remove or straighten one area of anatomy from another (Fig. 5–4).

1. Why do all radiographic images demonstrate distortion?

2. List the four types of radiographic distortion.

3. The most effective way to reduce motion from a radiographic image is to:
   a. Use restraints on the patient
   b. Use a high mAs technique
   c. Use a fast time
   d. Use a low kVp station

4. Which of the following techniques should offer a film with the least amount of motion unsharpness?
   a. 400 mA, 1/10 s, 60 kVp
   b. 200 mA, 0.2 s, 60 kVp
   c. 200 mA, 0.1 s, 69 kVp
   d. 400 mA, 0.05 s, 69 kVp

5. Which film will demonstrate the most geometric unsharpness? The least?
   a. 40-inch FFD, 6-inch OFD, 1-mm FSS
   b. 72-inch FFD, 10-inch OFD, 1.5-mm FSS
   c. 48-inch FFD, 4-inch OFD, .5-mm FSS
   d. 36-inch FFD, 4-inch OFD, .6-mm FSS

6. Radiographic film and intensifying screens cause _____ unsharpness.

7. Why do intensifying screens cause this unsharpness?

8. Parallax effect is most apparent when using _____.
   a. Thick films—perpendicular central ray
   b. Thin films—perpendicular central ray
   c. Thick films—angled central ray
   d. Thin films—angled central ray

9. Figure the radiographic image size of the following:
   a. 4-inch object, 40-inch FFD, 6-inch OFD
   b. 6-inch object, 72-inch FFD, 4-inch OFD

10. Figure the magnification factor for the objects in question 9.
    a.
    b.

11. Figure the percent of magnification for the objects in question 9.
    a.
    b.

12. Could you radiograph an 8 × 10-inch object and have the image fit on an 11 × 14-inch film using 40-inch FFD, 8-inch OFD?

13. How could you use shape distortion to your advantage when making radiographs?

LAB No. 1

Necessary Equipment

1. Energized x-ray room with two sizes of focal spot
2. Radiographic step wedge or penetrometer
3. Lead numbers (1/2-inch size)
4. 10 × 12-inch cassette with film
5. Processor
6. Lead rubber blocker

Place lead numbers on each step of the step wedge. Expose the step wedge twice by using an equal mAs, except for using the large focal spot size (FSS) for one and the small FSS for the second. Use equal FFD, collimation, and kVp. Process the film and examine it. The exposure with the small FSS should demonstrate more detail of the numbers than the one with the larger FSS. You should see a difference to a greater extent with the numbers on the higher steps.

LAB No. 2

Necessary Equipment

1. Energized x-ray room with two sizes of focal spot
2. Radiographic step wedge or penetrometer
3. Lead numbers (1/2-inch size)
4. 9.5 × 9.5-inch cassette with film
5. Nonscreen film in holder 8 × 10 inches
6. Processor

Place lead numbers on each step of the step wedge. Expose the step wedge with the screen film, then with the nonscreen film (make sure you use proper techniques). Check with your instructor. Inspect the films. You should be able to detect more detail on the nonscreen film.

LAB No. 3

Necessary Equipment

1. Energized x-ray room
2. Processor
3. Assorted radiolucent sponges
4. Radiopaque object (small bone-screw-calculator)

5. 9.5 × 9.5-inch cassette with film (2)
6. Ruler

Using the same object, expose it twice. First, use a 40-inch FFD and a 4-inch OFD. Second, use a 40-inch FFD and an 8-inch OFD. Before developing the films, figure the image size for each film. Process the films and check your figures. Notice how much more magification distortion is visualized on the film taken when the OFD is 8 inches.

Figure the percent of magnification for each film.

Figure the magnification factor for each film.

LAB No. 4

Necessary Equipment

1. Energized x-ray room
2. Processor
3. Assorted radiolucent sponges
4. Three quarters
5. 9.5 × 9.5-inch cassettes with film (3)
6. Ruler

Film no. 1. Place the three quarters on top of a cassette, 1 inch above each other (Fig. 5–5). Separate the quarters with sponges. Expose the film using perpendicular central ray.

Film no. 2. Use the same set-up, but angle the central ray by 30°.

Film no. 3. Use the same set-up. For this exposure, offset the central ray 8 inches from the coins (make sure the collimation is opened enough to cover the film). Use a perpendicular central ray for the exposure.

Develop the films.

Film no. 1: you will see one image if the coins are exactly superimposed.

Film no. 2: you will see three coin images because of the central ray angle (true distortion).

Film no. 3: you will see three coin images because of the divergence of the x-ray beam.

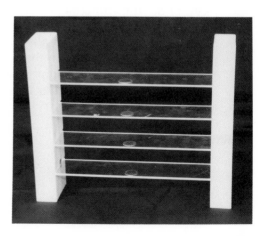

Fig. 5–5. A quarter box used to demonstrate distortion.

6

Radiographic Filters

OBJECTIVES *After completion, this chapter with the labs, the student radiographer should be able to:*

1. List and explain the three types of radiographic filters used in radiology departments.

2. Differentiate between a hardened and a softened x-ray beam.

3. State how the total x-ray tube filtration is figured.

4. State the National Council on Radiation Protection's total minimum x-ray tube filtration in aluminum equivalents below 50 kVp, at 50 to 70 kVp, and above 70 kVp.

5. Explain how to use the anode heel effect to advantage.

6. Discuss when additional compensating filtration might be used.

7. Take radiographs using various types of compensating filters.

The purpose of filters in radiography is to harden the x-ray beam. By using filtration, the x-ray beam undergoes some attenuation before it reaches the patient.

Any x-ray beam is heterogeneous; it has varying wavelengths. If you use a kVp of 80, the strongest wavelengths are 80 kVp; others will vary anywhere from 79 to about 30. Most of these low kVp photons never reach the film. If they do not reach the film, they cannot help with the formation of the image. What should be done with these photons? We should try to keep them from reaching the patient. When they reach the patient, they are too weak to pass through and are absorbed by the patient just under the skin.

INHERENT FILTRATION

All x-ray photons undergo some filtration because of how they are produced (Fig. 6–1).

The x-ray photons must get out of the glass tube, through the oil used for insulation, and past the collimator mirrors and plastic covering. Generally,

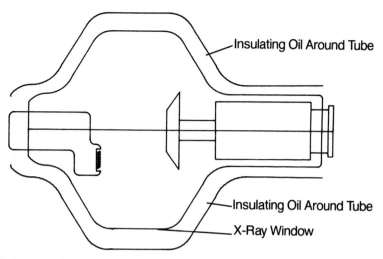

Insulating Oil Around Tube

Insulating Oil Around Tube

X-Ray Window

Fig. 6–1. Inherent filtration.

radiographers are not able to remove this type of filtration. It is called inherent filtration—inherent or always in the beam. Many of the weak x-ray photons do not reach the patient because they are absorbed by the inherent filtration. This type of filtration is tested and is measured in aluminum (Al) equivalent thickness. We know that it is not made of aluminum; however, if aluminum was used, it would be that thickness. Therefore, if inherent filtration is 0.75 mm Al equivalent, the glass, the oil, and the collimators attenuate the beam to the same extent as 0.75 mm of aluminum. (Some authorities refer to collimators as added filtration because the tube can operate without them.)

The National Council on Radiation Protection (NCRP) states certain requirements for operable radiographic machines:

	Total filtration must be a minimum of
Below 50 kVp	0.5 mm Al equivalent
50–70 kVp	1.5 mm Al equivalent
Above 70 kVp	2.5 mm Al equivalent

EXTERNAL (ADDED) FILTRATION

I am sure that the machines operating in your school are capable of generating kVp above 70. (An exception might be a unit used exclusively for mammography.) Therefore, the total filtration should be at least 2.5 mm Al equivalent. Most machines do not have inherent filtration to that level. To compensate, an added or external filter is placed between the x-ray beam and the patient. This added filter is most often made of aluminum (Fig. 6–2).

TOTAL FILTRATION

The capabilities of the inherent filter and the external filter together equal the total filtration. The total must be at least 2.5 mm Al equivalent (if the machine is capable of 70 kVp).

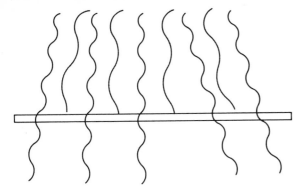

Fig. 6–2. Added aluminum filter removes the less penetrating or longer x-rays.

> 0.75 inherent
> + 2.0 added or external
> 2.75 Total filtration

In this example, the machine has more (0.25 mm) than the required amount of filtration. This excess is acceptable. A total of 2.25 mm Al equivalent is not acceptable. Let us work a problem.

Glass = 0.25 mm Al equivalent
Oil = 0.25 mm Al equivalent
Collimator = 0.25 mm Al equivalent
Added filter = 1.75 mm Al equivalent

Is this machine working under the guidelines of the NCRP?

> 0.25
> 0.25
> 0.25
> + 1.75
> 2.50 Total filtration

Yes, it does comply.

After performing labs for filtration, you can see that those little pieces of aluminum (Fig. 6–3) are worth their weight in "gold" for reducing the x-radiation dose to the patient.

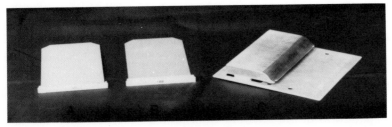

Fig. 6–3. A and **B,** External or added filters. **C,** Chest filter.

No disadvantage is associated with the use of filters. The radiographic density changes little by using more aluminum filtration. In many institutions, it is standard practice to use more than the required filtration to reduce even further the x-radiation dose to the patient.

After performing the lab for filtration, I think you will agree that the total filtration should be more than the minimum requirement of 2.5 mm Al equivalent.

COMPENSATING FILTERS

Another type of filtration used in radiography is compensation filtration. You know that all objects radiographed do not have the same density. Think of a patient who has heavy hips but relatively thin knees. If radiographing this patient's femur on a 14 × 17-inch film with one exposure, the knee area would have excessive density and the hip area would not have enough density. You could compensate for this difference by applying more exposure to the hip area and less exposure to the knee in several ways.

Anode Heel Effect

Anode heel effect is the variation of the intensity of the x-ray beam from the cathode to the anode side. The cathode side of the tube produces a beam with more strength than that generated on the anode side. The steeper the anode face angle, the greater the effect. An anode face angle of 11° produces more heel effect than that of a 17° face (Fig. 6–4).

The anode heel effect is less when increasing the focal-film distance (FFD), i.e., it is not apparent in radiographs of chests obtained with a 72-inch FFD. It does become evident as the FFD is decreased. An image produced at a 36-inch FFD on a 17-inch film demonstrates the heel effect. Most modern x-ray tubes have the anode and the cathode clearly marked so you can readily see which side is which. If you faced the patient mentioned previously (heavy hips and thin knees), place the patient on the table so the cathode side of the tube is over the hip area and the anode side is over the knee. You will be surprised at the results. The anode heel effect is usually used with success when radiographing the thoracic spine with the patient in the supine position (anterior projection). The anode heel effect is the most simple form of compensating filtration and should be used whenever you use a medium or short FFD.

Intensifying Screens as Compensating Filters

You probably know that intensifying screens are sold by speed. A faster screen needs less x-ray exposure than a slower screen for the same radiographic density. Therefore, we can use screens to our advantage to equalize the density of an image with a large difference in tissue density. A 14 × 17-inch cassette with a fast speed screen for the upper 14 × 8.5 inches and a

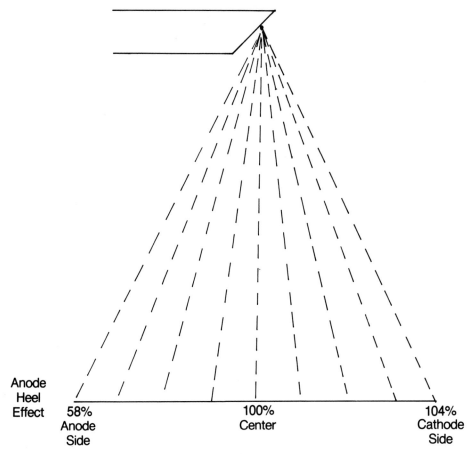

Fig. 6–4. Anode heel effect. X-ray intensity falls off toward the anode side of the x-ray tube.

Anode
Heel
Effect

58%
Anode
Side

100%
Center

104%
Cathode
Side

slower screen for the lower 14 × 8.5 inches (Fig. 6–5) could be used for patients that need compensation from one anatomic area to another on one film.

If a cassette of this nature is not available to you, there is another way to use screens as a compensating filter. Simply place a piece of paper in a portion

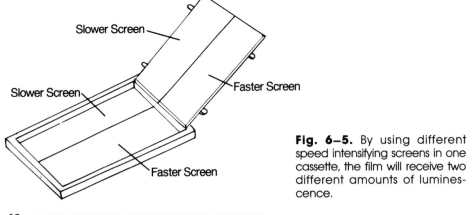

Slower Screen

Slower Screen

Faster Screen

Faster Screen

Fig. 6–5. By using different speed intensifying screens in one cassette, the film will receive two different amounts of luminescence.

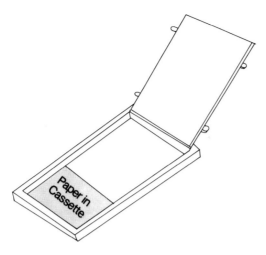

Fig. 6–6. By placing a sheet of plain paper in the cassette with the film, the film will receive less luminescence from the intensifying screen that is in contact with the paper.

of the screen between the film and the screen. The paper impedes the fluorescence of the screen and less light reaches the film (Fig. 6–6).

Wedge and Trough Filters

A wedge filter is shaped like a small ramp (Fig. 6–7). This type of filter is used in the same manner as the anode heel effect. The thicker portion of the filter is placed on the collimator to coincide with the less dense anatomic portion of the patient.

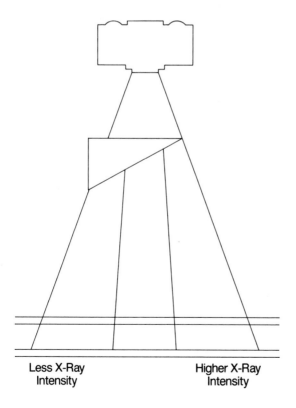

Less X-Ray
Intensity

Higher X-Ray
Intensity

Fig. 6–7. Wedge aluminum filter.

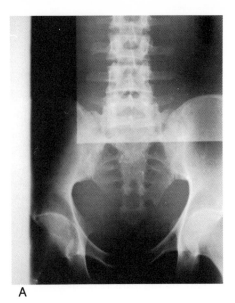
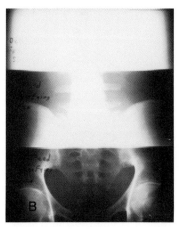

Fig. 6–8. A, Sheet of paper in cassette with film. **B,** Four different speed screens in one cassette.

A trough filter is smaller in the center than on both sides (Fig. 6–8). It is usually used in conjunction with chest radiographs. The purpose is to make the density of the radiograph somewhat equal for the lung tissue and the hilum area. The problem with using these types of filters is that they are attached to the bottom of the collimator and they obstruct the collimator light. A new filter is being manufactured, however, that is made of clear plastic impregnated with 30% lead. If a radiology department has a machine used principally to obtain chest radiographs, this type of trough filter could be used for most posteroanterior projections of the chest.

1. All x-ray beams are composed of _____ wavelength.
   a. Homogenous
   b. Hetergenous

2. Most very low kVp x-ray photons are absorbed by the _____.
   a. Cassette
   b. Radiographic film
   c. Patient skin
   d. Patient gonads

3. Inherent filtration consists of which of the following?
   1. X-ray tube window
   2. Oil for tube insulation
   3. Collimator
   4. Aluminum strip
   a. 1 and 2 only
   b. 1, 2, and 3 only
   c. 2, 3, and 4 only
   d. All the above

4. What is meant by total filtration of an x-ray beam?

5. What is the amount of total filtration necessary for an x-ray machine that has a kVp range of 40 to 140?

6. Why is compensation filtration used in radiology departments?

7. The x-ray beam is stronger or more penetrating on the _____ side of the x-ray tube.
   a. Cathode
   b. Anode

8. Anode heel effect is more noticeable on _____ FFD radiographs.
   a. Long
   b. Short

9. Which type of x-ray tube would demonstrate more anode heel effect?
   a. A chest tube used at a 72-inch FFD
   b. A 17° angle of anode face
   c. An 11° angle of anode face
   d. A 23° chest tube

10. Explain how intensifying screens could be used as compensating filters.

11. What is the difference between a wedge filter and a trough filter.

12. A trough filter would most probably be used for which of the following?
    a. Foot
    b. Knee
    c. Posteroanterior projection of chest
    d. Lateral projection of chest

LAB No. 1

Necessary Equipment

1. Energized x-ray room with removable added filter
2. Radiographic step wedge (penetrometer)
3. Processor
4. Assortment of aluminum filters
5. Rad check or dosimeter
6. 10 × 12-inch cassettes with film

Remove the added filter from the x-ray machine. Expose the step wedge and develop this film to determine if the technique is good. Using this same technique, expose a series of film portions increasing the added filtration by 0.5 mm until you reach 3 mm:

Film No. 1 no added filter
Film No. 2 0.5 mm Al added filter
Film No. 3 1.0 mm Al added filter
Film No. 4 1.5 mm Al added filter
Film No. 5 2.0 mm Al added filter
Film No. 6 2.5 mm Al added filter
Film No. 7 3.0 mm Al added filter

Develop these films. Set aside. Using the rad check or dosimeter, recreate the filter thickness amount and record the millirad for each exposure. Now compare the films with the millirad readings on a viewbox. You should notice that the film density does not change much but the amount of radiation increases significantly as the amount of filtration is decreased.

LAB No. 2 · DEMONSTRATION OF ANODE HEEL EFFECT

Necessary Equipment

1. Energized x-ray machine
2. Processor
3. 14 × 17 or 7 × 17-inch cassette filled
4. 2 equal density step wedges or 1 step wedge and sheet of lead rubber to cover one half of the cassette

If you have two step wedges, place one on the far edge of each side of the 17-inch side of the cassette. Using a 36-inch FFD, exactly center the cassette to the central ray and expose the step wedges. Somehow ascertain which side is the cathode and which side is the anode side. (I use a coin to determine anode side.) Use an exposure that will produce a less than normal density radiograph. Process the film and view it on the same 14 × 17-inch illuminator. The image of the step wedge on the anode side of the film will be less dense. If you try this process with a 72-inch or longer FFD, you probably will not see a difference (remember the anode heel effect is more noticeable with short FFD).

To perform this lab with only one step wedge, place the cassette in the direct center of the collimator. Place the lead rubber over one half of the cassette. Place the step wedge on the edge of the other side of the cassette. Expose the film, leaving the collimation at 14 × 17 inches. Now switch the step wedge with the lead rubber and repeat the exposure, making sure that the second exposure is the same as the first. Again, designate one side as either cathode or anode. Process the film. The results should be the same as the above (anode side will demonstrate less density than cathode side).

LAB No. 3 · PAPER AS A COMPENSATING FILTER

Necessary Equipment

1. Energized x-ray machine
2. Processor
3. 14 × 17-inch hinged cassette filled (1) (not daylight)
4. Sheet of paper, 14 × 8.5 inches
5. X-ray phantom (skull-abdomen-knee)

In a dark room, place the sheet of paper in the cassette so it fills one half of the area inside the cassette (make sure it also has unexposed film). Place the phantom in the center of the cassette on the radiographic table. Expose the phantom with normal technique. Process the film. The area of the phantom image on the half with the paper will be less dense than the other areas.

▬ 7

Radiographic Grids

OBJECTIVES   *After completion of this chapter with the labs, the student radiographer should be able to:*

1. Explain why grids must be used in radiographs.

2. List and explain the three main types of grids used in radiology departments.

3. List materials used in the construction of radiographic grids.

4. Explain causes for grid cut-off. List ways to correct grid cut-off.

5. Define grid radius.

6. Define grid ratio.

7. Define grid frequency.

8. Figure radiographic exposure techniques when changing from one grid ratio to another or from nongrid techniques to grid techniques.

The grid was invented in 1913 by Gustave Bucky. Before this time, it was not possible to radiograph large areas of the body with any degree of detail or contrast. The reason for this limitation was that too much of the scattered and secondary radiation reached the film.

X-rays, by their very nature, produce scattered and secondary radiation. The larger the area or the greater the x-ray exposure, the more scattered and secondary x-radiation produced. The problem with this scattered and secondary x-radiation is that it covers up the detail of the radiograph. With this in mind, you can see that if some of this scattered and secondary x-radiation was kept away from the film, the detail of the film would be better. The radiologist would be able to get more information from the film, thus enabling him or her to interpret the film more easily. One of the best ways to eliminate scattered and secondary x-radiation from reaching the film is the use of grids (Fig. 7–1).

Radiographic grids are devices constructed to absorb x-radiation before it reaches the film. Their purpose is to allow the remnant rays from the primary

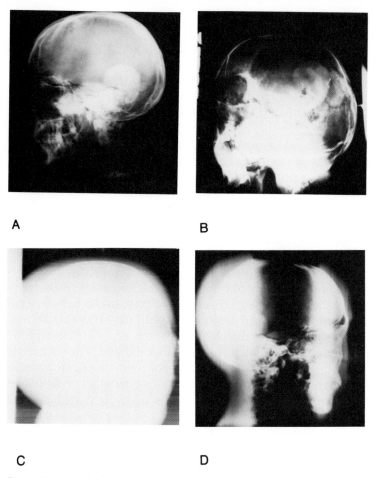

Fig. 7–1. Film of the skull phantom taken with a grid. **A,** Perpendicular central ray. **B,** 35° angle of central ray along the grid lines. **C,** 35° angle of central ray against the grid lines. **D,** Upside-down focused grid central ray perpendicular.

beam to pass through the grid, but those caused by scattered and secondary x-radiation are absorbed by the lead within the grid.

GRID CONSTRUCTION

Grids are thin lead strips placed between strips of some type of radiolucent material, such as cardboard or plastic. Because the primary remnant is stronger than the scattered and secondary remnant, more primary rays are able to pass through the grid; less scattered and secondary radiation gets through and it is absorbed by the grid. As a general rule of thumb, grids should be used for any part of the anatomy that measures 12 cm or more, with the exception of the lungs. (Remember, the lungs are the least dense organs in the body.) For this reason, most radiographic tables are equipped with grids. Many portable x-ray examinations also incorporate the use of a grid.

TYPES OF GRIDS

Three types of grids are available (Fig. 7–2):

1. Linear or parallel grids
2. Focused grids
3. Cross-hatch or criss-cross grids

In the linear or parallel grid, all the strips stand on edge, perpendicular to the height of the grid. This construction always allows for some grid cut-off, because the primary x-ray beam diverges from the source.

The focused grid is the most common type found in radiographic tables, because a standard focal-film distance (FFD) is used. The lead strips of this type of grid are angled from the center to the outside borders to accommodate for the divergence of the x-ray beam (Fig. 7–3). Because of these angled strips, focused grids have specific FFD ranges. They are sold with a recommended range, i.e., 48 to 72 inches or 35 to 45 inches. Because of the focus of these grids, proper use should prevent any grid cut-off. If the central ray is pitched across the table or angled across the grid, major cut-off occurs. When the recommended ranges are disregarded, grid cut-off occurs because the angle of the lead strips does not match that of the x-ray beam. In addition, when the central ray does not match the center of the grid, cut-off occurs (Fig. 7–4).

The cross-hatch grid is effective for removing large amounts of scattered and secondary radiation. It is actually two parallel grids placed on top of each other and oriented so that the strips are at right angles. The biggest drawback to the criss-cross or cross-hatch grid is that the central ray cannot be angled in either direction. For this reason, these types of grids can be used only with a perpendicular central ray. Usually, they are used only when the kVp is high.

GRID RATIO

All grids are sold with a specific grid ratio. Grid ratio is the ratio of the height of the lead strips to the distance between these lead strips (Fig. 7–5).

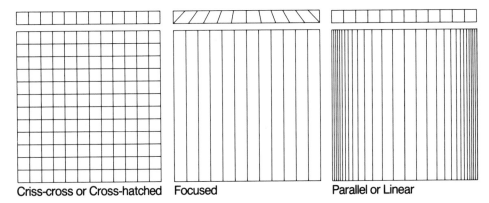

Criss-cross or Cross-hatched   Focused   Parallel or Linear

Fig. 7–2. The three most common types of grids used in radiography.

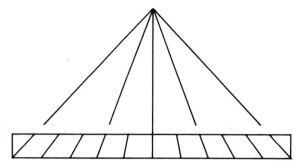

Fig. 7–3. Focused grid with central ray correctly aligned with lead strips.

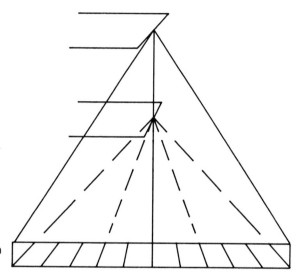

Fig. 7–4. Focused grid with central ray misaligned to grid.

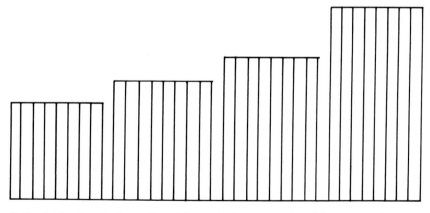

Fig. 7–5. Grid ratio. As the ratio of the grid increases, the thickness of the grid also increases, unless the space between the lead is reduced.

$$\text{Grid ratio} = \frac{h}{D}$$

Let us figure a grid ratio of this grid (grid A):

Height of lead strip = 1 mm

Space between strips = 0.1 mm

$$\frac{1}{0.1} = 10$$

Grid ratio = 10:1

Suppose the height of the lead strips in another grid (grid B) is reduced by one half:

Height of lead strips = 0.5 mm

Space between strips = 0.1 mm

$$\frac{0.5 \text{ mm}}{0.1 \text{ mm}} = 5$$

Grid ratio = 5:1

Now suppose the height of the lead strips in grid C is one half that in grid A and the space between them is reduced to one half the distance:

Height of lead strips = 0.5 mm

Space between strips = 0.05 mm

$$\frac{0.5}{0.05} = 10$$

Grid ratio = 10:1

Do you see how grids A and C have the same grid ratio? Grid B has a different ratio because the relationship between the height of the strips and the distance between them has changed.

GRID FREQUENCY

Grids are also manufactured with numerous numbers of lines per inch. This is also referred to as grid frequency. The more lines per inch in a grid, the less offensive the resulting film for the radiologist to interpret. Many lines tend to blend together, but a few lines per inch stand out more clearly in the radiographic image.

Figure 7–6 represents sections of grids used for teaching purposes. These sections have equal grid ratios but different grid frequencies. One has 60 lines

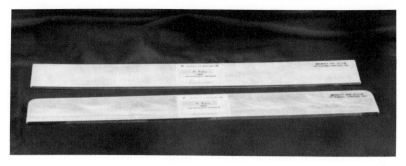

Fig. 7–6. Teaching grids. These grid strips assist with teaching grid ratio and grid radius.

per inch and the other has 80 lines per inch. The resulting radiographs have an equal density, but the lines are more visible on the 60-line grid image than on the 80-line image.

Naturally, the more lines per inch in a grid, the more difficult it is to manufacture, which means this type of grid costs more. Also, the more lines per inch, the thinner the grid must be to maintain the grid ratio.

Suppose grid A contains 100 lines per inch and grid B contains 60 lines per inch. If both grids have an 8:1 ratio, the ratio of height and distance must remain constant to maintain the 8:1 ratio. If you crowd more lines per inch of lead in an area, the space between each strip is reduced, thus changing the ratio. Therefore, to maintain a constant ratio, the more lines per inch, the thinner the grid. If the grid becomes too thin, it is less efficient for two reasons: (1) Too much of the scattered and secondary radiation passes through the grid, adding more fog to the film and covering up detail; and (2) It is less durable and warps easily. A warped grid is useless, because it adds artifacts to the radiograph.

A few things to remember when working with grids.

1. All grid techniques increase patient dose when compared to a nongrid technique.
2. As the grid ratio increases, so does the patient dose of x-radiation.
3. All nonmoving grids cause grid lines on the radiographs.
4. As the grid ratio increases, the radiographs increase in contrast (high contrast-short scale contrast). As contrast increases, the visible radiographic detail increases.
5. All radiographs taken with the Bucky grid have a loss of detail because of the increased object-film distance.
6. The central ray can always be angled in the same direction as the lead strips, but it cannot be angled against the strips (except for a criss-cross grid, which allows no angle).
7. Some grids are manufactured into cassettes. Do not use these cassettes in conjunction with the Potter Bucky.
8. Radiographic grids are expensive and should be treated with respect.
9. Low ratio grids, such as 5:1 or 6:1, are used in fluoroscopy units because the image area is usually small, i.e., 1/4 of a 9.5 × 9.5 = 2.375 × 2.375, which is only 4.75 square inches of area.

Whenever a grid is used for radiography, the amount of x-ray exposure must be increased. The reason for this increase is that some of the x-radiation is absorbed by the grid, so it does not reach the radiographic film. Any nongrid technique can be adapted to a grid technique. The grid ratio is the determining factor for this technique change. The following is a list of the most common ratio grids and the changes needed for each:

5:1 grid ratio: nongrid mAs technique × 2
6:1 grid ratio: nongrid mAs technique × 3
8:1 grid ratio: nongrid mAs technique × 4
12:1 grid ratio: nongrid mAs technique × 5
16:1 grid ratio: nongrid mAs technique × 6

The knee is a part of the anatomy for which some radiology departments select a grid technique and some use a nongrid technique. Let us convert some techniques for such radiographs.

A nongrid technique to image the knee is 2 mAs, 68 kVp, 40-inch FFD. You want to use a Bucky grid. The grid ratio for this particular table is 12:1. What is the new technique for this knee?

2 mAs × 5 = 10 mAs

New technique = 10 mAs, 68 kVp, 40-inch FFD

Another case involves the Bucky technique to image a knee with a 16:1 grid, which is 18 mAs, 62 kVp, 40-inch FFD. You find out that the patient is pregnant. The physician still wants the radiograph, so you decide to radiograph this knee using a nongrid technique to save the patient from as much radiation as possible.

18 mAs ÷ 6 = 3

New technique = 3 mAs, 62 kVp, 40-inch FFD, nongrid

You can use 3 mAs instead of 18, a savings of 15 mAs per knee exposure. How could you reduce the x-ray exposure even further? Use the 15% kVp rule. Instead of using 3 mAs, 62 kVp, increase the kVp by 15% to 71 and cut the mAs to 1.5. You can see how previous chapters help you as well as your patients!

Let us change from one grid to another. The technique is 20 mAs, 66 kVp, 8:1 grid. The goal is to keep the density equal but to use a 5:1 grid.

I find the most accurate method for this type of problem is to take the technique back to nongrid.

8:1 grid factor = 4

20 ÷ 4 = 5 (nongrid technique)

5 × 2 = 5:1 factor

New technique = 10 mAs, 66 kVp, 5:1 grid

You could also work this problem by subtracting the 8:1 grid factor from the 5:1 factor, which is 2, and then dividing the original 20 by 2, equaling 10. It seems that sometimes this grid change becomes a problem of whether to divide or to multiply. Most radiography students find it easier to go back to the nongrid technique. So, first divide and then multiply.

Additional grid radiographic exposure problems when working with grids follow.

PROBLEM 1: A knee was radiographed in the radiology department using the following factors:

40-inch FFD
66 kVp
12:1 grid
200 mA
1/20 s

The patient was admitted to the hospital and placed in traction because of a fracture. You must figure the radiographic technique for the portable examination. You have a 6:1 grid and you must use a 32-inch FFD because of the traction. What should you use for mAs to keep the density equal?

New FFD = 32
kVp = 66
Grid ratio = 6:1
mAs?

1. Figure original mAs. 200 × 1/20 = 10
2. Change to nongrid technique. 10 ÷ 5 = 2
3. Figure inverse square law to change 40-inch to 32-inch FFD: 1.28
4. 1.28 is nongrid technique. Change to 6:1 grid ratio: 1.28 × 3 = 3.84
5. If you could use 3.84 mAs, the portable technique would be equal to the original technique (Note: the new film will have more magnification).

You probably cannot get 3.84 mAs on the portable machine, but use an mAs that is as close as possible and the technique will be fine, i.e., use 3.5 or 4 mAs.

PROBLEM 2: A good radiographic technique for a cervical spine is:

72-inch FFD
Nongrid
80 kVp
300 mA
50 ms

The radiographs demonstrate too much fog and you want to use an 8:1 ratio grid. What time should you use with the 600 mA station?

1. Figure original mAs. 300 × 0.05 = 15 mAs
2. Multiply nongrid mAs by 4. 15 × 4 = 60
3. 600 × ? = 60
4. 60 ÷ 600 = 0.1s or 100 ms

PROBLEM 3: A shoulder radiograph is usually taken with the following factors:

40-inch FFD
8:1 grid
72 kVp
100 mA
1/20 s

How do you lengthen the scale of contrast and use a 12:1 grid?

1. Figure original mAs. 100 × 1/20 = 5 mAs
2. Change 5 mAs to nongrid. 5 ÷ 4 = 1.25
3. Multiply nongrid mAs by 5. 1.25 × 5 = 6.25
4. Change kVp to 83. 15% of 72 = 11
5. Change mAs to 3.125 to compensate for increased kVp
6. Use 83 kVp, 3 mAs, 40-inch FFD, 12:1 grid for equal radiographic density

PROBLEM 4: A radiograph of the abdomen was obtained in the radiology department by using:

300 mA
1/10 s
77 kVp
40-inch FFD
12:1 grid

The examination must be repeated, but you must use a portable machine that has only a 100 mA station. What time should you use for this radiograph if you are using a 6:1 grid and 65 kVp?

1. Figure original mAs. 300 × 1/10 = 30
2. Figure nongrid technique. 30 ÷ 5 = 6
3. 15% of 77 = 12, so if you use 65 kVp, mAs must be doubled. 6 × 2 = 12
4. 12 is nongrid technique. Change to 6:1 grid ratio: 12 × 3 = 36
5. 36 is new mAs; 100 ÷ 36 = 0.36
6. 0.36 is the new time (use time as close to 0.36 as possible)

1. Who invented the grid?

2. Scattered and secondary radiation obscures which of the following?
   a. Contrast   b. Detail   c. Density

3. Radiographic grids limit the amount of x-radiation reaching:
   a. The film   c. The technologist
   b. The patient   d. Both a and b

4. Grids should be used with anatomic areas that measure more than _____ cm of thickness.
   a. 4   b. 8   c. 12   d. 16

5. List the three types of grids.

6. Which type of grid is usually found in radiographic tables?

7. What is meant by grid frequency?

8. Usually a criss-cross grid is used in conjunction with which of the following:
   a. Only angled central ray films   c. Low kVp, high mAs techniques
   b. Very high mAs techniques   d. High kVp techniques

9. What is grid ratio?

10. If two grids have equal ratios and one has 110 lines per inch and the other has 80 lines per inch, which grid is thinner?

11. As the grid ratio increases, the radiographic contrast _____.
    a. Increases   b. Decreases   c. Remains the same

12. A 6:1 grid technique is 600 mA, 30 ms. What mAs should you use if you switch to a nongrid technique?

13. Figure the new technique for the following:
    a. 300 mA   300 mA
        1/10 s   ? s
        68 kVp   78 kVp
        8:1 grid   16:1 grid
    b. 400 mA   ? mA
        50 ms   100 ms
        90 kVp   77 kVp
        12:1 grid   5:1 grid
    c. 60 mAs   ? MAS
        80 kVp   92 kVp
        40-inch FFD   60-inch FFD
        8:1 grid   16:1 grid

LAB No. 1 · GRID RATIO

Necessary Equipment

1. Energized x-ray room
2. Processor
3. X-ray phantom (abdomen is best)
4. Various ratio grids (6:1, 8:1, 12:1)
5. 14 × 17-inch cassettes filled (4)

Radiograph the phantom using a nongrid technique. Ascertain from your clinical instructor that it is a good technique. Figure the grid technique for each grid using your nongrid technique. Use mAs as your variable (page 52). Using the new techniques, expose the phantom with each grid, making sure that each can be identified after processing. Process the films and mount on a viewbox bank in order from nongrid film to the highest ratio film. Notice how much more scattered and secondary radiation is absorbed as the grid ratio increases. You should notice that all the films have approximately the same density. The contrast increases as the ratio increases.

LAB No. 2 · GRID CUT-OFF (ANGLED CENTRAL RAY)

Necessary Equipment

1. Energized x-ray room
2. Processor
3. X-ray skull phantom
4. 10 × 12-inch cassettes filled (3)
5. 10 × 12-inch 8:1 ratio parallel or focused grid

Place the phantom in the anteroposterior position on the cassette covered with the grid. Using a perpendicular central ray, expose the skull (film no. 1).

With the second film, set up the phantom in the same way, except angle the central ray with the grid lines 30° caudad. Expose the skull using the same technique (film no. 2).

Using the third cassette, set up the phantom as for film nos. 1 and 2, except angle the central ray against the grid lines (turn the grid in the other direction). Expose the skull using the same technique (film no. 3). Process all three films. Film nos. 1 and 2 should have approximately the same density. Film no. 1 might be darker; because of the 30° angle in film 2, the central ray has more to go through when it is angled on a skull). Film no. 3 demonstrates only a shadow of the skull, because the central ray was angled at the grid lines and was absorbed almost entirely by the lead in the grid.

LAB No. 3 · GRID CUT-OFF (IMPROPER GRID FREQUENCY)

Necessary Equipment

1. Energized x-ray room
2. Processor
3. X-ray skull phantom
4. 10 × 12-inch cassette filled (3)
5. 10 × 12-inch grid with 40-inch focus (8:1 or 12:1 ratio)

Radiograph the phantom in the lateral position with a 40-inch FFD using a normal radiographic technique (film no. 1). Ascertain from your clinical instructor that it is a good technique.

Figure a technique for a 20-inch FFD and expose the phantom with the second cassette. Use the grid (film no. 2).

Figure a radiographic technique for a 60-inch FFD and expose the phantom with the third cassette (film no. 3).

Process all three films and check the results. Film no. 1 will have grid lines, but they should not be obstructive to the eye. View the film at about a 25-inch distance from your pupils. Film no. 2 will have a large amount of cut-off because of how the diverged x-ray beam struck the grid lines. (This film will also demonstrate a great deal of magnification owing to the short FFD). Film no. 3 will demonstrate a slight amount of grid cut-off because of the increase in the FFD. Film no. 3 looks better than film no. 2 because the image magnification is reduced in film no. 3.

8

Intensifying Screens

OBJECTIVES *After completion of this chapter with the labs, the student radiographer should be able to:*

1. Define the following terms as they pertain to radiography:
   a. Luminescence
   b. Phosphorescence
   c. Fluorescence
   d. Spectral matching

2. Discuss how an intensifying screen converts the x-radiation into the latent image.

3. List and explain the layers of an intensifying screen.

4. Discuss differences between calcium tungstate and rare earth crystals when used as intensifying screens.

5. Work mAs problems using the intensifying factor of screens.

6. Work radiographic technique factors when changing from one intensifying screen speed to another or from nonscreen techniques to screen techniques.

7. Discuss radiographic detail factors involved with using certain intensifying screens.

8. Discuss patient dose to x-radiation when using faster versus slower intensifying screens.

9. Define poor film screen contact.

10. Make radiographic exposures to check for poor film screen contact.

Nothing in the history of radiography, with the exception of the x-ray tube, has had as big an impact as the invention of the intensifying screen. The fluorescent intensifying screen was invented by Thomas A. Edison in 1896. The function of the intensifying screen is to convert the x-ray beam into visible fluorescent light. It is this light that exposes the radiographic film. If the entire image is formed by the use of the x-ray beam, more x-radiation is needed to produce the image. Whenever screens are used, the greater part of the image is formed by light. If this is true, how does it happen? Most cassettes use double screens and double-sided emulsion film. When the x-ray beam excites the screens, they in turn fluoresce or glow. This fluorescence is in direct proportion to how much radiation passes through the object or patient.

The use of intensifying screens changes the density of the film a great deal. You cannot go from department to department and figure radiographic techniques if you do not know the speed of the screens that are used. A few years ago, screens were sold with names such as High Speed, Par Speed, and Detail Speed. Things are a bit easier to work with now, because they are sold with numbers ranging from 50 to 800. These numbers represent the speed of the screens. It is also possible to change the speed of some screens by the type of film that is used in conjunction with that screen.

SCREEN LUMINESCENCE

The term luminescence is used when working with intensifying screens. Luminescence is defined as the ability to emit light with stimulation. This phenomenon assumes two types: *fluorescence* and *phosphorescence.* When an object demonstrates fluorescence, it does so only during stimulation (faster than 10^{-8} second; an object that demonstrates phosphorescence does so less rapidly. It begins to glow after stimulation begins (slower than 10^{-8} second). Such an object continues to glow after the stimulus has ceased. Which type of luminescence should be used in conjunction with intensifying screens? Fluorescence, because the screens stop glowing as soon as the x-ray exposure is terminated. If intensifying screens demonstrate phosphorescence, they continue to glow after the exposure stops. This would cause the radiographic film to become fogged. Phosphorescence is a good attribute for fluoroscopy screens used in radiology departments, because the screen demonstrates a visible image after the radiologist has released the exposure switch. Try to remember which type of luminescence is used for each type exposure:

Fluoroscopy screens—Phosphorescent

Intensifying screens—Fluorescent

SCREEN CONSTRUCTION

Intensifying screens are extremely expensive and require care to preserve their life. The construction of screens helps them to last longer (Fig. 8–1).

The base layer is the bottom layer in relation to the film and is the support for the rest of the screen. It is usually made of cardboard or plastic. This base layer must be flexible, because flexible cassettes are available (usually used for knees and shoulders).

The next layer is called the reflective layer, which is used to direct the light photons toward the film. The fluorescence from the active layer of the screen spreads out in all directions. The shiny reflective layer changes the direction of the light photons traveling away from the film and aims them toward the film, thereby increasing the speed of the screen.

The most important layer of the screen is the active or phosphor layer—the layer that glows when stimulated by the x-ray exposure. This phosphor layer

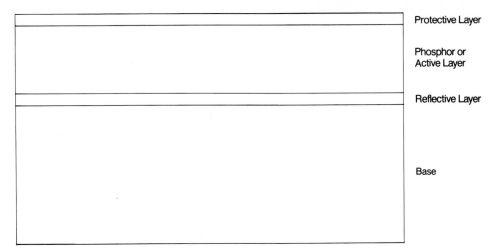

	Protective Layer
	Phosphor or Active Layer
	Reflective Layer
	Base

Fig. 8—1. Cross-section of an intensifying screen.

converts the x-ray photons into visible light. The color of that visible light has become important in the past few years. From 1896 until about 1970, all intensifying screens were made of calcium tungstate or barium lead sulfate. These compounds fluoresce to a blue-violet color. Therefore, screen film was manufactured to be sensitive to this color range. This spectral matching was not a problem, because all screen films were sensitive to blue-violet.

With the newer rare earth screens (see page 60), however, the speed of the active layer of the screen depends on the size of the phosphor crystals and the thickness of the phosphor layer. The thicker the layer, the faster the screen. A thick layer fluoresces more brightly than a thin layer. The larger the phosphor crystal size, the faster the screen (Fig. 8—2). A larger crystal absorbs more x-ray photons. If they absorb more, they emit more light. Some manufacturers use standard size crystals and vary the phosphor thickness to change the screen speed.

The layer that touches the radiographic film is the protective layer. It is usually a thin coating of transparent plastic covering the phosphor layer to protect the screen from scratches. This layer also helps to prevent static electricity. When screens are cleaned, this layer is the only area that is touched.

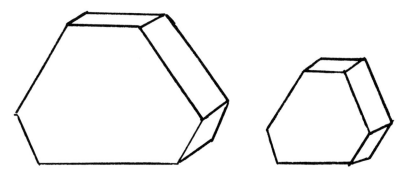

Fig. 8—2. Larger crystals increase intensifying screen speed.

RARE EARTH SCREENS

The newer rare earth screens are being used in place of the calcium tungstate screens because of their speed. The rare earth screens are approximately twice as fast as those made of calcium tungstate, with no loss of detail. With this new type of screen, the patient dose is decreased by at least one half. When the patient dose is less, the life of the x-ray tube is usually longer. When the patient dose is reduced, it is usually possible to reduce the exposure time and, therefore, the incidence of motion on the films is also reduced.

The reason that these rare earth screens are faster is because they absorb more x-ray photons and are able to convert this absorption into more light. They are problematic in that most rare earth screens do not fluoresce to the blue-violet range. Films must be manufactured with the ability to be matched with blue-green or green range. Most radiology departments in large health facilities have incorporated the use of rare earth screens.

The rare earth phospors that are in use at this time are gadolinium and lanthanum. Both of these rare earth elements glow in the green range when used independently. If activated by terbium as a phosphor, lanthanum emits color in the blue-violet range.*

INTENSIFYING FACTOR

How much will an intensifying screen change the density of a radiographic film? The answer depends on the screen type and speed. If you know the radiographic exposure needed with and without screens, you can figure the intensifying factor of a particular screen with this formula.

$$\text{Intensifying Factor} = \frac{\text{Exposure without screens}}{\text{Exposure with screens}}$$

$$\frac{60 \text{ mAs (no screens)}}{2 \text{ mAs (with screens)}}$$

$$60 \div 2 = 30$$

The intensifying factor of this screen is 30.

SCREEN RADIOGRAPHIC TECHNIQUE

Let us figure a technique to use for a nonscreen film if you know the intensifying factor of a certain screen. If the intensifying factor is 42 and the exposure with screens is 1.5 mAs:

---

*Selman, J: *The Fundamentals of X-Ray and Radium Physics.* 7th ed. Springfield, IL, Charles C Thomas, 1985.

$$42 = \frac{?}{1.5}$$

$$42 \times 1.5 = 63$$

If you must use a nonscreen film (maybe a foreign body extremity), you should use 63 mAs instead of 1.5. You probably will have to use either 60 or 65. You can see that when using nonscreen radiography, the patient receives considerably more x-radiation.

You must be thinking that all radiographic films should be taken with intensifying screens. This practice, of course, saves the patient from excessive x-radiation. I am sure that you have noticed that most films are taken with a film/screen combination. Sometimes, however, detail is of utmost importance, and this is when the nonscreen films are used. The entire image derives from direct x-ray exposure exciting the film. The detail is better and there is more latitude for error when using nonscreen techniques; more technique is used to image the film. Nonscreen films have a longer scale of contrast than screen films. When discussing screen/film combinations, the lower the number, the longer the scale of contrast.

Place the following in order, beginning at the longest scale of contrast:

a. 800 film/screen (F/S) combination
b. 100 F/S combination
c. 200 F/S combination
d. 50 F/S combination
e. Nonscreen film/direct exposure film
Answer: e, d, b, c, a

The same answer applies for the amount of x-radiation the patient receives. The lower the film/screen (F/S) combination, the more x-radiation the patient receives.

In most radiology departments, the same combinations are used for most radiographic examinations. Some departments, however, incorporate different speeds for different examinations.

Suppose an 800 F/S system is used for pediatric and emergency room patients, a 400 F/S system for routine department work, and a 200 F/S system for detail work, such as arthrograms and detail extremity work.

Assume the routine technique for a knee in the department is

10 mAs
40-inch FFD
64 kVp (12 cm)
400 F/S combination
12:1 Bucky grid

What technique will offer equal density if the same patient comes to the emergency room and you must use an 800 F/S system? The 800 F/S system is twice as fast as the 400 F/S system, so all you have to do is divide the mAs by 2. Use 5 mAs and leave everything else the same. When one system has twice the speed as another, you need one half the technique. You can see that the easiest way to do this is to change the mAs. You could also use any of the following to obtain films of equal density when using the technique just described.

A. 5 mAs
   40-inch FFD
   64 kVp
   800 F/S combination—screens 2 times faster
   12:1 Bucky grid
B. 10 mAs
   40-inch FFD
   54 kVp—15% rule
   800 F/S combination—screens 2 times faster
   12:1 Bucky grid
C. 2 mAs
   40-inch FFD
   54 kVp—15% rule
   800 F/S combination—screens 2 times faster
   Nongrid—12:1 grid ÷ mAs by 5
D. 2.5 mAs
   40-inch FFD
   74 kVp—15% rule
   800 F/S combination
   12:1 Bucky grid

These five techniques offer approximately equal density on the radiograph of the knee. If, however, we compare the four films to the original, we will see some differences. Film A will have a shorter scale of contrast because the 800 F/S system increases the short scale of contrast. Film B will have a shorter scale of contrast because (1) the kVp is lower by 15% and (2) the 800 F/S system increases the short scale of contrast. Film C will have a shorter scale of contrast because (1) the kVp is lower by 15% and (2) the 800 F/S system increases the short scale of contrast. The overall difference will probably be of a longer scale because of the removal of the grid. This nongrid technique produces less patient exposure. Film D will have longer scale of contrast because of the increase of 15% kVp, but it will have a shorter scale because of the change of the film/screen combination. This film will probably have a scale of contrast most like that of the original film, because the increase of kVp is offset by the faster film/screen combination.

If you want to change to a lower film/screen combination to gain detail on certain films, the preceding technique works the same in reverse. Using the same original knee technique, change to a 200 F/S combination because the radiologist needs more detail. The 200 F/S combination has one half the speed of the original 400 F/S system, so you need two times as much radiation. You could use any of the following:

A. 20 mAs—2 times mAs
   40-inch FFD
   64 kVp
   200 F/S combination
   12:1 grid

B. 10 mAs
   40-inch FFD
   74 kVp—15% increase
   200 F/S combination
   12:1 grid
C. 4 mAs
   40-inch FFD
   64 kVp
   200 F/S combination
   Nongrid ÷ mAs by 5
D. 2 mAs
   40-inch FFD
   74 kVp—increase by 15%
   Nongrid ÷ mAs by 5 after changing to 10 because of 15% kVp

I do not recommend the use of a nongrid technique when using over 70 kVp, but it can be done when reduced x-radiation is important.

Look at the following and determine which would be most dense:

20 mAs	20 mAs	5 mAs
80 kVp	68 kVp	92 kVp
6:1 grid	Nongrid	8:1 grid
200 F/S combination	100 F/S combination	400 F/S combination

First, get rid of the grids:

6.6 mAs	20 mAs	1.25 mAs
80 kVp	68 kVp	92 kVp
÷ mAs by 3	Nongrid	÷ mAs by 4
200 F/S combination	100 F/S combination	400 F/S combination

Next, equalize kVp (I would change all to 80):

6.6 mAs	10 mAs	2.5 mAs
80 kVp	68 − 80 makes mAs 10	92 − 80 makes mAs 2.5
200 F/S combination	100 F/S combination	400 F/S combination

Now, equalize the screens (I would use the 100 F/S combination as the base):

| 12.2 | 10 | 10 |
| mAs × 2 | 100 | mAs × 4 |

When everything is equalized, B and C have equal density and A is the most dense. When you first look at the four factors of each technique, it is difficult to know which is the most dense. When you work the problem step by step, it is easy to figure which is which.

Whenever intensifying screens are used, some detail is lost. One thing cannot be emphasized enough when working with screens: they must be mounted in the cassette so film screen *contact* is good. This means that the film must touch the screens on both sides with equal pressure on all areas. Good film screen contact is harder to maintain with larger size cassettes. Poor screen

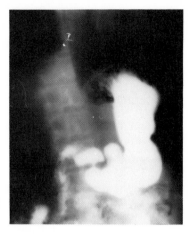

Fig. 8–3. Radiograph of the stomach with poor film screen contact.

contact is usually demonstrated at or near the center of the film (Fig. 8–3). Poor screen contact is many times confused with patient motion.

To check screens for film screen contact, use the wire mesh test (Fig. 8–4). A wire mesh embedded in lucite is placed on the cassette containing the film in question. Take a radiographic exposure of the wire mesh and develop the film. If poor film screen contact exists, the image appears fuzzy in the poor screen film contact area.

Intensifying screens should be cleaned periodically. Any dirt or dust on the screens appears as light artifacts on the film because the fluorescence is hindered by the dirt and is not as bright to that area of the radiographic film. Take care not to scratch or mar the screen surface, because any unremovable marks on a screen render that screen useless. Screen manufacturers sell cleaning fluid to use with their screens, and you should follow the directions of these manufacturers in its use.

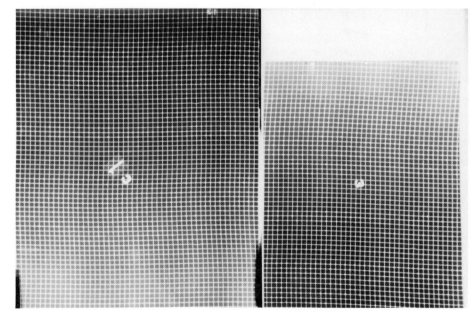

Fig. 8–4. Radiograph of wire mesh to check for screen contact.

1. The intensifying screen was invented by _____.

2. When working with intensifying screens, the radiographic image is formed mostly by:
   a. Action of x-rays
   b. Light produced by fluorescence
   c. Light produced by phosphorescence
   d. Luminescence in the form of phosphorescence

3. It would benefit the patient if a fluoroscopy screen is able to phosphoresce.
   ( ) True   ( ) False
   Why?

4. List the layers of an intensifying screen from top to bottom.

5. The reflective layer of a screen should make that screen _____.
   a. Faster   b. Slower
   Why?

6. The phospor layer of a screen converts x-ray photons to _____.

7. What is meant by spectral matching?

8. The speed of the active layer depends on crystal _____ and crystal _____.

9. The newer type rare earth screens are replacing the calcium tungstate because of _____.

10. Figure the intensifying factor for the following:
    a. Nonscreen technique = 66 mAs
       Screen technique   = 2.5 mAs
    b. Nonscreen technique = 120 mAs
       Screen technique   = 5 mAs

11. If an intensifying screen has an intensifying factor of 42, what technique should you use for a nonscreen technique if you use 0.7 mAs for a screen technique?

12. The main disadvantage of screen radiography over nonscreen radiography is _____.

13. Figure an equal density radiographic technique for the following:

Original Technique	New Technique
a. 20 mAs	? mAs
80 kVp	92 kVp
400 F/S combination	800 F/S combination
40-inch FFD	40-inch FFD

b. 15 mAs
   66 kVp
   200 F/S combination
   40-inch FFD

? mAs
56 kVp
400 F/S combination
40-inch FFD

c. 10 mAs
   70 kVp
   400 F/S combination
   8:1 grid
   40-inch FFD

200 mA
? s
80 kVp
100 F/S combination
12:1 grid
40-inch FFD

LABS

LAB No. 1 • *OBSERVATION OF SCREEN FLUORESCENCE*

Necessary Equipment

1. Energized radiographic room
2. Calcium tungstate intensifying screen
3. Rare earth intensifying screen (green spectrum)

Open the cassette on the radiographic table. Center the tube to the screen and open collimation to cover the screen. Turn off the lights. While exposing the screen, look through the window at the fluorescence. The calcium tungstate screen should fluoresce to a blue-violet color. Repeat using the rare earth screen. Notice the fluorescence is now green.

LAB No. 2 • *RADIOGRAPHIC TECHNIQUES USING DIFFERENT INTENSIFYING SCREEN SPEEDS*

Necessary Equipment

1. Energized radiographic room
2. 200 F/S combination cassette filled (2)
3. 400 F/S combination cassette filled (2)
4. Radiographic step wedge

Radiograph the step wedge with the same technique using the 200 F/S and then the 400 F/S combinations. Process the films. The 400 F/S combination film should have twice the radiographic density as the 200 F/S combination.

    Next use two different techniques; use twice the mAs for the 200 system as you use for the 400 system. Process the films. They should exhibit equal density. The 400 F/S system film will have a shorter scale of radiographic contrast.

LAB No. 3 • DEMONSTRATION OF FILM SCREEN CONTACT

Necessary Equipment

1. Energized radiographic room
2. Old 14 × 17-inch cassette with intensifying screens (not one that is used in department) filled
3. Smooth block of wood 1/2 to 3/4 inches thick, about 2 inches long, and 2 inches wide
4. X-ray phantom or a couple of dried bones

In a dark room, place wood in the cassette with film. Close the cassette. Radiograph phantom or bones and process the film. The area around the wood should have a fuzzy appearance that resembles motion. You know that the objects were not moving—you are looking at poor screen contact.

■ 9

Radiographic Film

OBJECTIVES *After completion of this chapter with the labs, the student radiographer should be able to:*

1. List and explain the layers of a radiographic film.

2. Discuss film/screen combination and why it is important to radiography.

3. Define the characteristics of radiography film that are important to the radiographer.

4. Discuss when radiography film with extremely long scale contrast should be used.

5. Define crossover radiation.

6. Discuss ways to eliminate static from radiographs.

Modern radiographic film is manufactured using some of the highest standards of quality control. It is extremely rare to purchase a box of radiographic film that contains defects. Originally, x-ray images were recorded on glass plates. These, of course, were fragile, heavy, and hard to store. Imagine an x-ray series containing 8 to 10 films made of 8 to 10 separate panes of glass!

CONSTRUCTION

Doubled-sided emulsion films have seven layers (Fig. 9–1). These films have no right or wrong side. Starting at one side, thse layers are as follows: *protective coat, emulsion, adhesive layer, base, adhesive layer, emulsion,* and the other *protective coat.* Single emulsion film is manufactured for specialty areas, such as units used only for chest radiography, in which only one screen is employed, or for use in single-screen mammography units. These films have only four layers and must be placed in the cassette with the emulsion side toward the screen.

The protective layer of the film is composed of a thin covering of tough gelatin over the emulsion layer. This covering allows the film to travel through the processor rollers without getting scratched. It also prevents fingerprints and marks from fingernails from altering the films.

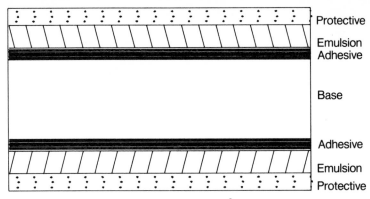

Fig. 9–1. Cross-section of double-sided emulsion film.

The emulsion layer is the most important layer of the film. The emulsion is the sensitive area of the film that is responsible for the radiographic image. Emulsion is produced by the method of combining silver with gelatin. The emulsion is spread evenly, usually, on both sides of the polyester base.

The adhesive layer of the film is placed on the film to ensure that the emulsion does not peel away from the base. This layer must be transparent so it will not detract from the detail of the image.

The film *base* is the thickest portion of the radiographic film. It is also the support structure of the film. Since the early 1960s, film bases have been made of polyester. Polyester has two distinct advantages as the base material: (1) it is strong and durable, and (2) it does not burn with an open flame. It is a relatively easy process to manufacture polyester into specific thicknesses to be used in film production. Most manufacturers of radiographic film use a blue dye in the film base. The purpose is so the films do not cause so much eye strain for the radiologists. You can see this blue tint readily on processed films that have collimation lines or on films that have been processed without an x-ray exposure.

CHARACTERISTICS

The speed of a particular film depends on the size of the crystals and the thickness of the crystal layer. The larger the crystals, the faster the film. A consequence of this increased speed, however, is that the film demonstrates a loss of detail. Also, the thicker the crystal layer, the faster the film, although again, a loss of detail occurs.

The emulsion of radiographic film is produced to be sensitive either to the action of x-ray photons or to visible light. About 99% of radiographic film is used in conjunction with intensifying screens. This film is sensitive to either blue-violet or the green range of color. It is extremely important to use the correct film/screen combination. The other type of film (nonscreen) is more sensitive to x-ray photons. This type of film must be used for direct exposure; it should never be used with screens because the film is not as sensitive to the color spectrum and this color will detract from the film's detail. This nonscreen film image is produced only by the action of the x-rays and the radiographer must use significantly more radiation to the anatomic part to obtain an equal density film. Nonscreen film is used only when detail is paramount; for example, for a lateral projection of the nose and for imaging extremities when the presence of a foreign body is suspected.

The most important film characteristics from the radiographer's viewpoint is film speed and film latitude. The speed was discussed in part previously. It has a lot to do with what type of intensifying screens are used in the health facility. The faster the film, the less radiation needed to produce a radiograph. A faster film may be the film of choice if working in a pediatric hospital, because most of the time you are dealing with both somatic and genetic radiation. Film latitude is of great importance because it deals with two main aspects: (1) the scale of contrast, and (2) the amount of leeway for error in the radiographic technique. With no room for error in technique, I am sure the result would be a lot more repeat films! Too much latitude, however, and the films tend to look flat and the detail is hard to see.

Some films are manufactured to have exceptionally long scale contrast. In most instances, these films are used for chest radiographs. If the films have a long scale of contrast, it is possible (with high kVp) to visualize both the lungs and the mediastinal area with the same radiographic exposure. In some health facilities, radiographers use this long scale-type film with kVp values as high as 150. If this type of film is used for areas that usually are imaged with short scale contrast (such as extremities), the radiographic image will have long scale contrast that makes these films harder for the radiologist to interpret.

Single-sided emulsion films are sold for use when detail is important. These films are usually used in single-screen cassettes. The emulsion side of the film must be placed next to the intensifying screen. This type film is used for mammograms and also in industrial radiography. Single-emulsion film is sometimes used in conjunction with chest radiography. This practice is no longer common because use of the single-emulsion film is associated with a higher radiation dose.

Other radiographic films are found in radiology departments, including the following:

Roll film for spot radiography
Video film
Dental film
Panoramic film
Duplicating or solarization film
Subtraction film
16- or 35-mm cine film

Roll film is used for spot radiography in a 70- or 105-mm camera with image-intensified fluoroscopy. This film is usually sold in 150-foot rolls. Video film is used with the images produced from a cathode ray tube. Cathode ray tubes are used for computed tomography, ultrasonography, and magnetic resonance imaging.

For some of the new emulsion (T-Grain, Eastman Kodak, Rochester, NY) manufacturers use what is called flat crystals. These crystals have the advantage of allowing the films to trap more light without adding thickness to the emulsion. Therefore, these thinner films both are faster and produce films with greater detail (Fig. 9–2). This type of emulsion incorporates a magenta dye to

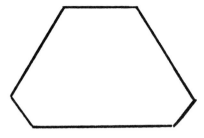

Fig. 9–2. Flat crystals. Films are thinner and faster when this type of crystal is used.

reduce crossover radiation. Crossover radiation, also called punch-through radiation, is the light from one screen through the film to the other screen. It causes the image to become fuzzy because of the divergence of the light photons. The presence of the magenta dye (red and blue mixed) inhibits the light from going all the way through the film and reaching the other screen.

Dental films, which are individually wrapped, are sold for use in the radiography of teeth or small body areas. Panoramic film is used to radiograph the entire dental arch on one sheet of film. It is usually used by dentists, orthodontists, and temporomandibular joint specialists. Duplication film is used when you must copy radiographs. Another name for this film is solarization film. Subtraction film is used in a technique by which you take away part of a film image, leaving vital information on the film. Cine film is used principally for heart catheterizations. Once developed, the film is viewed on a movie screen with the use of a motion picture projector.

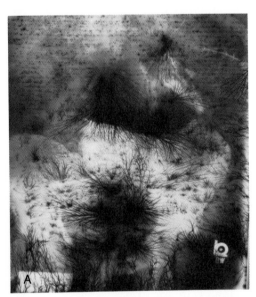
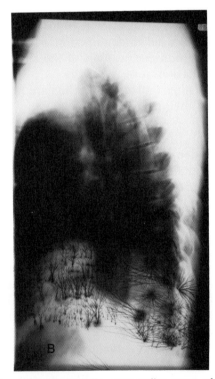

Fig. 9–3. A. Radiographic film of abdomen, demonstrating static over entire area of radiograph. **B.** Radiograph of lateral thoracic spine with static over lower portion of film.

Ensuring high-quality radiographs requires care of the radiographic films. All photographic films are manufactured with expiration dates. Films usually have about an 18-month expiration period. Radiographic film should be used before 1 year is left to the expiration date; for example, if the expiration date is December, 1991, try to use the film by December, 1990. Old films begin to deteriorate, decreasing both detail and contrast. Unused radiographic films should be stored on edge in a cool, dry place away from any radiation source. If radiographic film boxes are stacked, pressure static may be evident on the films (Fig. 9–3). Static may also result if the relative humidity is too low (below 40%). The ideal humidity in which to store films is 40 to 60%; above 60%, they may swell and become sticky. Heat is another enemy of radiographic films. Too much heat greatly reduces the contrast by adding fog to the films. The temperature in a storage area for radiographic films should not be higher than 68° F.

1. List the seven layers of a double-sided radiographic film.

2. Which of these layers is the thickest?

3. How does crystal size affect film speed?

4. The faster the radiographic film the _____ the image produces.
   a. More detail   b. Less detail

5. Radiographic films used in conjunction with intensifying screens are more sensitive to:
   1. X-ray photons
   2. Blue-violet luminescence
   3. Green luminescence
   a. All of the above   b. 1 and 2   c. 1 and 3   d. 2 and 3

6. What is the chief disadvantage of using nonscreen film?

7. What is meant by film latitude?

8. Why would a film be manufactured with exceptionally long scale contrast?
   This film would be an asset when used for _____.
   a. Extremities   b. Gastrointestinal series   c. Chest   d. Spine
                              with barium

9. Single-sided emulsion films would benefit which of the following radiographic examinations?
   a. Breast   b. Abdomen   c. Knees

10. Name at least four of the less often used radiographic films found in radiology departments.

11. Video radiographic film is used for what purpose in a radiology department?

12. What are two important advantages to using polyester as the base material for radiographic film?

13. All radiographic films are manufactured with _____.
    1. Expiration dates
    2. Double-sided emulsion
    3. Blue dye in the base
    4. T-Grain crystals
       a. All of the above   b. 1 only   c. 1, 3, and 4   d. 2, 3, and 4

14. Radiographic films should be stored on edge.
    ( ) True   ( ) False

15. Radiographic films that have been exposed to high temperatures demonstrate _____.
    a. Spots   b. Static   c. Fog   d. More detail

16. Radiographic films should be stored in a relative humidity of _____.
   a. 10–12%   b. 20–40%   c. 40–60%   d. 60–80%

LABS

LAB **No. 1**

Necessary Equipment

1. Energized x-ray room
2. Processor
3. Cassettes with calcium tungstate screens
4. Cassettes with green emitter rare earth phospors
5. Radiographic films; green-sensitive, blue-violet-sensitive, and non-screen type
6. Radiographic phantom
7. Rad check or other radiation exposure rate device

Steps

1: Radiograph the phantom with a proper film/screen combination using the correct radiographic technique

2: Radiograph the phantom with the nonscreen film using the correct radiographic technique (nonscreen)

3: Place a sheet of nonscreen film in a cassette and expose it using a proper technique for that screen

4: Place a sheet of blue-sensitive film in a green emitter cassette and expose using a proper technique for that cassette

5: Using a rad check machine or other radiation exposure rate device, check the amount of radiation for each exposure

Compare the radiation exposures and the radiographic films. Film no. 1 should have proper density and a relatively low x-radiation dose. Film no. 2 should have proper density, long scale contrast, and an extremely high dose of x-radiation. Film no. 3 should have insufficient density but the same x-radiation as film no. 1. The wrong film was in the cassette. The film was more sensitive to x-ray photons but was exposed by visible light from the screens in the cassette. Film no. 4 also possesses insufficient density because the film was sensitive to blue-violet but the screen was fluorescing in the green range. You can see that by comparing these results, it is important to choose the proper film with the proper screen type and to remember that when you choose to use a nonscreen film, the patient dose of x-radiation is higher than when you use intensifying screens.

◢ *10*

Beam-Restricting Devices

OBJECTIVES *After completion of this chapter with the labs, the student radiographer should be able to:*

1. List and explain five ways that radiographic quality is compromised by not using proper collimation.

2. Define stem or off-focus radiation and how collimators remove this radiation.

3. Discuss why four-sided collimation on radiographs is helpful to the radiographer.

4. Discuss reasons for using a radiographic cone or cylinder to further reduce the field size.

5. Figure field size coverage for a cone or cylinder.

6. State the purpose of a radiographic aperture diaphragm.

7. Figure the opening size for a radiographic aperture diaphragm for various field sizes.

8. Discuss when lead blockers should be used in radiography.

COLLIMATORS

As you know, x-rays cause scattered and secondary radiation. The larger the area of the x-ray beam, the greater the amount of scattered and secondary radiation produced. This radiation detracts from the image. It covers up the detail of the image and adds to the density of the film. The use of close collimation is one of the best ways to improve the detail of any radiographic image. With the invention of the variable collimator and the application of these collimators on all x-ray units, there is no excuse for not using close collimation on all films. Any technologist that does not use good collimation does five things that detract from a good radiographic image:

1. Cover up detail
2. Increase film density
3. Increase patient exposure to x-radiation

4. Increase your own exposure
5. Make the radiographs more difficult to interpret

Modern collimators are easy to operate (Fig. 10–1). They are manufactured with specific focal-film distance (FFD) settings that correspond to inch or centimeter settings. The collimator works with four main lead shutters that open and close with two knobs on the face of the collimator. One knob is for cross shutters and the other is for longitudinal shutters. These knobs are rotated to the desired position by the technologist. Collimators shed light on the patient and are used as positioning guides for technologists. The light is produced by a bulb located in the back of the collimator and the light is focused by mirrors so it does not interfere with the image. These mirrors do attenuate the beam somewhat and are considered part of the inherent filtration of the machine. Protruding from the top of the collimator is another series of shutters that absorb the stem or off-focus radiation before it reaches the patient or the film. The bottom of a collimator usually has a sheet of plastic with both a crosswise and a longitudinal black line used for centering the tube to the film.

It is always a good idea to produce radiographs that have a collimated edge on all four sides. When a technologist follows this procedure, any x-radiation exposure to portions not on the film is not possible, i.e., when a technologist radiographs a chest, the lens of the eyes should never be in the primary beam. Collimation on the top of the film ensures that the lens of the eyes is not in the primary beam.

CONES AND CYLINDERS

All diagnostic medical x-ray machines, with the exception of dental units, must be equipped with collimators. To limit the scattered and secondary ra-

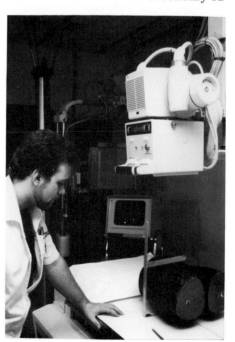

Fig. 10–1. Collimator is located under the x-ray tube structure.

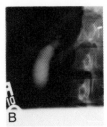

Fig. 10–2. Radiographs of the gallbladder after a fatty meal. Notice the detail of the ducts.

A   B

diation further, the use of cones and cylinders is recommended for certain examinations. I think cones should always be used for studies of the paranasal sinuses and the gallbladder (Fig. 10–2). You can probably think of others. Cones are especially useful for radiographic examinations in which collimation extends past the anatomic region being radiographed. A good example is a lateral radiograph of the nose. The cone absorbs some of the x-rays that otherwise would scatter back onto the outside portion of the nose, thus covering up some of the detail.

Most cones have a round bottom; however, they can be made in any shape. Before collimators were used, many departments had rectangular cones, because the shape of the film is rectangular.

When using a cone, you are able to figure out how much radiographic film area is covered by using this formula:

$$\text{Film size} = \frac{\text{Size of cone at bottom} \times \text{FFD}}{\text{Target to bottom of cone}}$$

Suppose you want to cover an area 9 inches in diameter. You have a 3-inch diameter cone. You want to use a 40-inch FFD. The distance from the target to the bottom of the cone is 12 inches.

$$\text{Film size} = \frac{3 \times 40}{12}$$

$$\frac{120}{12}$$

Film image diameter = 10 inches

Notice what happens when you change one factor. Ten inches is too large. Change the FFD to 36 inches.

$$\text{Film size} = \frac{3 \times 36}{12}$$

$$\frac{108}{12}$$

Film image diameter = 9 inches

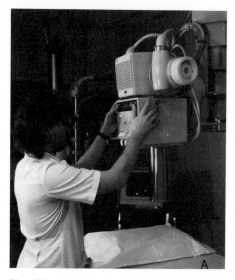 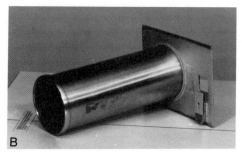

Fig. 10–3. A, Radiographic cylinder attached to the collimator. **B,** Cylinder for use in conjunction with a collimator.

In some departments, radiographers use cones in conjunction with existing collimators, but most use cylinders. Cylinders are an adaptation of a cone; they are tubular instead of flared like a cone (Fig. 10–3). Many cylinders have a mechanism that enables them to be either extended or collapsed. Cylinders are usually attached directly under the collimator. Whenever a cylinder is used, the collimation should be adjusted to just cover the area inside the cylinder. This adjustment helps to remove the off-focus or stem radiation. The use of cylinders improves the detail of "spot" films (Fig. 10–4).

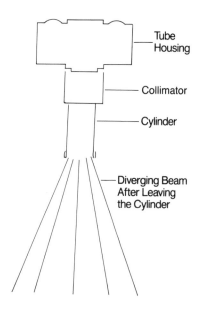

Fig. 10–4.

APERTURE DIAPHRAGMS

Another way to limit the size of the x-ray beam and thus improve detail is by the use of an aperture diaphragm. This device is placed between the tube and the film (Fig. 10–5). For machines without collimators, it is placed under the added filter. If you are using a machine equipped with a collimator, an aperture diaphragm is placed under the plastic on the bottom of the collimator. Aperture diaphragms can also be placed in the fluoroscopy unit for use during such procedures as a knee or shoulder arthrogram. Image detail is enhanced because the diaphragm absorbs some scattered and secondary radiation.

Aperture diaphragms are made of either lead or stainless steel. Most departments use stainless steel diaphragms because steel is not as malleable as lead.

To figure out how large the opening in the diaphragm should be, you must know the following:

1. FFD
2. Field size (image size)
3. Target distance to placement of diaphragm

When you determine these variables, put them into this formula:

$$\text{Aperture diaphragm size} = \frac{\text{Field size} \times \text{Target to diaphragm placement}}{\text{FFD}}$$

Let us figure:

$$\frac{(10 \times 12) \times 12}{40}$$

$$\frac{10 \times 12}{40}$$

$$\frac{120}{40} = 3$$

$$\frac{12 \times 12}{40}$$

$$\frac{144}{40} = 3.6$$

A diaphragm that has an opening that is 3 inches by 3.6 inches would produce a 10 × 12-inch image if the FFD was 40 inches and it was placed 12 inches below the target of the x-ray tube. If you have a diaphragm and you want to know how large an area it would cover at a specific FFD, just substitute variables in the formula, as follows:

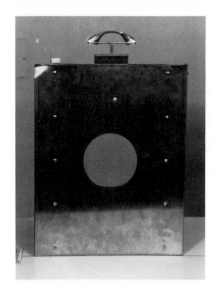

Fig. 10–5. Diaphragm used for imaging the skull.

$$(3 \times 3.6) = \frac{(? \times ?) \times 12}{40}$$

$$(3 \times 3.6) \times 40 = (120 \times 144)$$

$$120 \div 40 = 3$$

$$144 \div 40 = 3.6$$

An aperture diaphragm that measures 3 × 3.6 would cover an area of 10 × 12 with an FFD of 40 inches and the diaphragm was 12 inches from the target of the x-ray tube. It is possible that a set of collimators is stuck in the fully open position. You might be able to use this collimator if you make diaphragms from lead strips and tape them under the collimator. This method should be used only for short periods of time until the collimator can be repaired.

LEAD BLOCKERS

Pieces of lead rubber found in radiology departments are of great value when good detail is important (and it is always important). I am sure lead rubber sheets are used in most departments when more than one exposure is made on a single cassette. They also come in handy for absorbing scattered and secondary radiation and not allowing it to reach the film (Fig. 10–6). In numerous radiographic examinations, a piece of lead rubber can enhance the radiographic image. The following is a partial list of examinations for which the use of lead blockers is valuable:

1. Shoulder (Fig. 10–7)
2. Clavicle
3. Lateral projection of knee (Fig. 10–8)

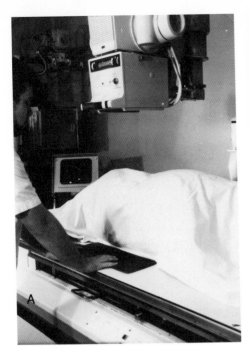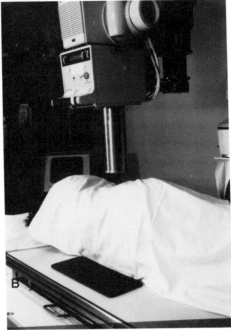

Fig. 10–6. A, Lead blocker to pick up scattered and secondary radiation. **B,** Lead blocker plus cylinder absorb more scattered and secondary radiation.

  4. Lateral projection of thoracic spine
  5. Lateral projection of lumbar spine (Fig. 10–9)
  6. Lateral projection of sacrum and coccyx
  7. Lateral projection of facial bones
  8. Anteroposterior and lateral projections of feet (Fig. 10–10)
  9. Lateral projection of scapula
 10. Lateral projection of sternum

Because of the entrance of the central ray to the body part in these examinations, x-ray coverage occurs in areas where no anatomy exists. These areas are where the lead is placed. The use of lead becomes even more important

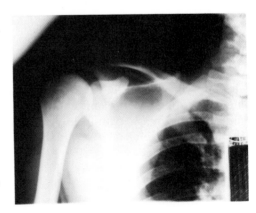

Fig. 10–7. Anteroposterior projection of the shoulder.

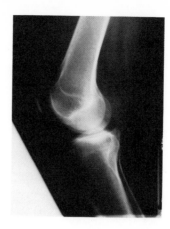

Fig. 10–8. Lateral projection of the knee.

when using higher kVp. The lead absorbs the greater amounts of scattered and secondary radiation that are produced by higher kVp. Try to remember this the next time you radiograph any of the regions just mentioned.

Excess field coverage contributes to the overall film density. Any film taken with a large area of coverage has more density relative to one taken with a small area of coverage because of more scattered and secondary x-radiation. Some students find this concept hard to understand. When the x-ray beam is collimated to a smaller area, the beam is not more concentrated. Much of the scattered and secondary radiation is eliminated because it is not produced. It is set up mainly in the patient, and when the patient area is smaller owing to close collimation, scattered and secondary radiation is not produced. Therefore, when an area is reduced in size in order to keep equal density on the film images, the technique must be increased. Suggested technique changes for film size changes follow:

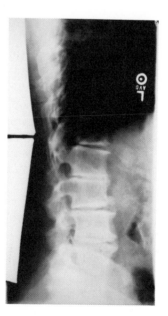

Fig. 10–9. Lateral projection of the lumbar spine.

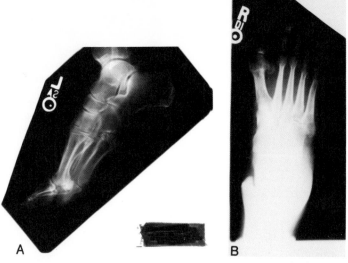

Fig. 10–10. Lateral (**A**) and anteroposterior (**B**) projections of the foot.

Field Size		
From	To	mAs Increase
14 × 17 inches	11 × 14 inches	About 10%
35 × 43 cm	25 × 35 cm	
14 × 17 inches	10 × 12 inches	About 20%
35 × 43 cm	25 × 30 cm	
14 × 17 inches	8 × 10 inches	About 30%
35 × 43 cm	20 × 25 cm	
14 × 17 inches	5 × 7 inches	About 50%
35 × 43 cm	12.7 × 17.7 cm	

These changes also work in reverse. If you must change from a small field size to a larger one, you must decrease the technique by approximately the same percent.

Work this problem. The technique for a 14 × 17-inch abdomen film was 30 mAs, 66 kVp, 40-inch FFD. What, if any, changes should be made if you must now do a coned film of the gallbladder area (8 × 10 inch) in the same position?

Increase the mAs by about 30%. Use 9 more mAs than the original technique, mAs of 39. You probably will have to use 40. The density of the second film will be equal to the first, yet the second film will have more detail because more scattered and secondary radiation has been removed from the radiographic image.

Now, work one problem in reverse. A 5 × 7-inch spot film of the lumbar spine (L2 and 3) was taken using 50 mAs, 72 kVp, 40-inch FFD. What, if any, changes should be made if you must radiograph the entire abdomen to evaluate the abdominal anatomy in the same position?

Decrease the mAs by 50%. Use 25 mAs less for the 14 × 17-inch field size. You should use 25 mAs and the two films will have equal density. Notice that the coned-down film has more detail than the larger film.

Many student radiographers have difficulty with this concept because more and more radiography rooms and departments are equipped with automatic exposure control devices. These devices automatically terminate the exposure when the film has received enough radiation to reach a predetermined density. Because of this setting, equal density is maintained when the collimation is changed. Sometimes, the use of these automatic exposure control devices is confusing to student radiographers. (The devices are discussed in more detail in Chapter 13.)

Remember that only a lazy or noncaring radiographer uses less collimation than should be used. In doing so, he or she is adding to the patient's dose of radiation and is making the films harder for the radiologist to interpret. I am of the opinion that all films should have four-sided collimation. What do you think? Why?

1. List the five things that detract from the image of a film that is not closely collimated.

2. A modern collimator usually works with _____ main lead shutters.
   - a. 1
   - b. 2
   - c. 3
   - d. 4

3. The light bulb is located _____ the collimator shutters.
   - a. In front of
   - b. Behind
   - c. Inside

4. The light is focused on the patient by the use of _____.
   - 1. Collimator shutters
   - 2. X-ray beam
   - 3. Mirrors
   - a. 1 only
   - b. 2 only
   - c. 3 only
   - d. All the above

5. The upper portion of the collimator has a series of shutters used to remove the _____.
   - 1. Stem radiation
   - 2. Off-focus radiation
   - 3. Remnant radiation
   - a. 1 only
   - b. 2 only
   - c. 3 only
   - d. 1 and 2

6. Could the following size cone be used to cover a field size of 9 × 9 inches with these factors?
   - a. Cone size of 2.5 × 2.5 inches
   - b. 40-inch FFD
   - c. 14-inch distance from target to bottom of cone

7. What size aperture diaphragm opening would be needed for the following:
   - a. 40-inch FFD
     Field size of 9 × 9 inch
     Target to diameter placement of 16 inches
   - b. 72-inch FFD
     Field size of 13 × 16 inches
     Target to diameter placement of 14 inches.

8. Explain why it is a good idea to use a lead blocker on the radiographic table when performing a lateral lumbar spine radiograph and why one is not needed when performing the posterior view?

9. What changes would you make in this technique of a pelvis exposed on a 14 × 17-inch film if you had to take a coned-down exposure of the left sacroiliac articulation on an 8 × 10-inch film?

LAB No. 1 • *EXCESSIVE DENSITY BY UNDER COLLIMATION*

Necessary Equipment

1. Energized radiographic room (do not use the phototimer)
2. Processor
3. Abdomen phantom
4. 14 × 17-inch cassettes filled (3)

Using the same radiographic technique, expose the phantom by using three separate exposures. Film no. 1: use 14 × 17-inch collimation. Film no. 2: use 8 × 10-inch collimation. Film no. 3: use 5 × 7-inch collimation. Compare the density of each film after they are processed.

LAB No. 2 • *IMPROVEMENT OF CONTRAST BY THE USE OF COLLIMATION*

Necessary Equipment

1. Energized radiographic room (do not use the phototimer)
2. Processor
3. Abdomen phantom
4. 14 × 17-inch cassettes filled (3)

Expose the first film by using a 14 × 17-inch collimation. Check this film to make sure the technique is good. Expose the next film by using a 10 × 12-inch collimation and increase the mAs by 20%. Lastly, expose a film using an 8 × 10-inch collimation and increase the mAs by 30%. After the films are processed, check them for contrast and density. The film density should be about the same, but the contrast should show improvement on the last two films. (This difference is more apparent when working with "real" patients because of the body fluid.)

LAB No. 3 • *FIELD SIZE COVERAGE*

Necessary Equipment

1. Energized radiographic room
2. Processor
3. Cone or cylinder
4. X-ray phantom
5. 14 × 17-inch cassette filled

Using a predetermined FFD, figure the field size for the cone you are using. Expose the radiographic phantom, process the film, and measure the image. Does the measurement coincide with your figures?

LAB No. 4 • *MAKING A RADIOGRAPHIC APERTURE DIAPHRAGM*

Necessary Equipment

1. Energized radiographic room
2. Processor
3. At least four small strips of lead rubber
4. Tape or glue
5. X-ray phantom
6. 10 × 12-inch cassette filled

Figure out the diaphragm opening for a field size of 7 × 9 inches using a 40-inch FFD. Tape or glue the lead strips to this size opening. Attach the strips under the plastic on the collimator and expose the radiographic phantom. Process the film and measure the field size. Does it coincide with the 7 × 9 inches?

LAB No. 5 • *REDUCTION OF SCATTERED AND SECONDARY RADIATION BY USE OF A LEAD BLOCKER*

Necessary Equipment

1. Energized x-ray room
2. Processor
3. Two lead rubber blockers
4. Abdomen phantom
5. 14 × 17-inch cassettes filled (2)

Place the phantom on the table in the lateral position and center the lumbar-sacral region to the center of the table. Collimate to about 8 × 17 inches. Expose the first film using at least 85 kVp. Before exposing the second film, place the lead rubber blockers close to the posterior portion of the phantom. Expose the second film. Process the films and compare the amount of scattered and secondary radiation on the two films. Look closely at the spinous processes and notice the greater contrast on the film taken with the use of lead blockers.

11

Geriatric and Pediatric Radiography

OBJECTIVES *After completion of this chapter, the student radiographer should be able to:*

1. Recognize that the geriatric patient usually suffers from more pathologic conditions than young adults.

2. List problems from the standpoint of radiography when dealing with the geriatric patient.

3. To make compensations in radiographic exposure techniques for the geriatric patient.

4. Recognize that the pediatric patient presents certain problems to the radiographer.

5. Group pediatric patients by their age and/or size for proper radiographic exposure techniques.

6. To make changes in exposure techniques for the pediatric patient in radiography.

7. Deal effectively with the problem of motion on radiographs of pediatric patients.

Many patient factors come into play when figuring radiographic techniques. Some patients have tissue that is more dense than others. More and more, radiographers are working on geriatric patients. The population of the United States is aging and will continue to age for quite a few more years. Problems arise concerning technique factors when radiographing the elderly. The incidence of pathologic conditions is higher in this group of patients than in younger adults. Therefore, consider the following:

1. Many elderly women suffer from osteoporosis (most common in the Caucasian race).
2. Many elderly have poor muscle tone (disuse, atrophy).
3. Many elderly suffer from hearing loss.
4. Many elderly suffer from poor eyesight.

5. It is sometimes more difficult to get the elderly into proper radiographic positions.
6. Many times, patient restraints must be used for the elderly.

I am quite sure that you have been involved in helping to radiograph elderly patients. You have probably been amazed by the age of some of the patients. Some look much older than the requisition states and many look much younger. Many things are involved in the aging process and many times the calendar years do not mean much. Often, it is not much more than a good or bad judgment call when deciding what technique to use on an older patient. If the technique charts in your health facility are geared toward the young (45 years), healthy patient, some adjustments must be made to compensate for many of the older patients.

The most common difference between the older adult and the younger adult is the lack of muscle tone in the older patient. X-ray photons penetrate poor, weak muscles more easily than they do well-toned muscle tissue. Therefore, you can understand why many radiographic films of the elderly are overpenetrated.

When radiographing elderly patients that appear to have poor muscle tone, reduce the mAs by about 25 to 30%. I recommend that if a particular radiographic examination has four or more exposures, check the first film for "technique." This step is especially pertinent when a patient is suffering from osteoporosis. This disease is one that sometimes justifies reducing both the mAs and the kVp. When considering radiographic techniques for the elderly, you should try to use fast time, whether or not you are phototiming the examination (see Chapter 13). The short time is used because the elderly sometimes do not understand your instructions and many times they cannot hear your instructions. They also, many times, have difficulty remaining in the proper radiographic position and have a tendency to shake.

Elderly patients, like children, should never be left unattended in a radiographic room. It is also easy to injure an elderly patient. They usually have bones that are more brittle and they bruise easily.

Use extreme care when restraining the elderly. The restraints often put pressure on the wrists or ankles and it is quite possible to cause an abrasion of the skin with bleeding. In most cases, if this happens, an incident report must be submitted.

Let's work some problems. Use the following technique for an anteroposterior projection of the lumbar spine:

40 mAs
78 kVp
Patient measurement is 20 cm
40-inch FFD

An 88-year-old woman must have an anteroposterior projection of the lumbar spine. The patient's measurement is 18 cm. What radiographic technique should you use?

Subtract 25 to 30% mAs. 40 − 25 to 30% = 28–30 mAs
Patient measurement is 2 cm less. Reduce kVp to 74

(Make sure mAs is figured using a high mA station.)

The same patient has osteoporosis. What additional change in radiographic technique should you make?

Use 5 or 6 less kVp. 68–69 kVp instead of 74
Reduce the mAs as in preceding problem

The shoulder girdle is one of the regions of the body that is a challenge to a radiographer. If you usually radiograph the shoulder area of athletic patients and then are called on to radiograph the shoulder of an elderly patient, especially one that has little muscle tissue, you may find the first exposure is dark. It is important to think about each patient that you are called on to radiograph. I have seen shoulders that need only one quarter of the suggested radiographic technique for proper density. The little old lady from the area nursing home is a perfect example. Shoulder radiography is another situation that warrants checking your first exposure before going on with the examination. If you are going to work in a nursing home setting, you probably should make the technique charts to accommodate the elderly instead of the 45-year-old patient.

Pediatric patients also can cause problems for the radiographer. One fact to remember when making radiographic techniques for children is that they have a greater percent of water per body weight than adults. If more water is present in the body, scattering of the remnant x-ray photons is greater. Therefore, the radiographic techniques for children should be figured using less kVp than is used for adults.

Children usually are classified into three or four groups to the age of about 12 years. The following classification lists can be used as a guideline for pediatric radiographic techniques. It is hard to use age as a factor because many children are either large or small for their age.

CHART I

Grouped by 3		Grouped by 4	
Infant	Birth to 2.5 years	Infant	Birth to 1 year
Preschool	2.5 to 6 years	Baby	1 to 3 years
Grammar school	6 to 12 years	Preschool	3 to 7 years
		Grammar school	7 to 12 years

In most health facilities in which variable kVp techniques are used, radiographers group the children into the 3- or 4-group categories and use these or similar multiplication factors:

CHART II

Grouped by 3	Use
Birth to 30 months	0.3 × adult mAs
30 months to 6 years	0.5 × adult mAs
6 years to 12 years	0.75 × adult mAs
Grouped by 4	
Birth to 1 year	0.25 × adult mAs
1 year to 3 years	0.5 × adult mAs
3 years to 7 years	0.7 × adult mAs
7 years to 12 years	0.9 × adult mAs

For all the preceding techniques, you should measure the anatomic part and use the appropriate kVp (of course, the kVp is lower because the part is smaller).

Let us work some problems.

The technique for the pelvis in an adult is 20 mAs, 66 kVp if the pelvis measures 18 cm. What should you use on a child's pelvis? The child is 6 years old and the pelvis measures 10 cm (use the 4 group)?

Pelvis measures 8 cm less, so use 16 kVp less. 66 − 16 = 50 kVp
Age factor is 0.7. 20 × 0.7 = 14 mAs
Field size is reduced to 10 × 12-inch area. Add 20% to 14 mAs. 14 × 0.20 = 2.8. 2.8 + 14 = 16.8 mAs
Use 16.8 mAs at 50 kVp
New technique for equal density: 50 kVp, 16–18 mAs

The technique for a lateral skull film in an adult is 12 mAs, 64 kVp if the skull measures 14 cm. You must radiograph the skull of an 8-year-old child in the same position. The child's skull measures 11 cm in the lateral position (use group 3).

Patient's skull measures 3 cm less, so use 6 less kVp. 64 − 6 = 58 kVp
Age factor is 0.75. 12 × 0.75 = 9 mAs
No change is needed for collimation
New technique: 9 mAs, 58 kVp

If your health facility does not have technique charts for pediatric patients, all you need is a list of the age factors. This list will assist you in determining proper radiographic techniques.

Another aspect of pediatric radiography is the use of high mA techniques. A short exposure time is essential when radiographing children. Motion of both types (voluntary and involuntary) is a problem with pediatric patients. Children should be placed in restraining devices whenever possible (Figs. 11–1 and 11–2). Very young children are usually more content when they are secured and covered than when someone tries to hold them on a radiographic table (Fig. 11–3).

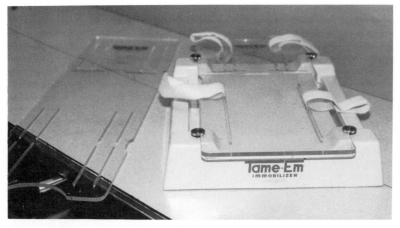

Fig. 11–1. Immobilizer for infants.

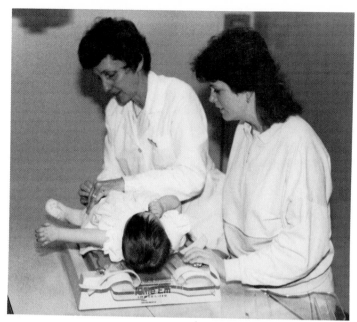

Fig. 11–2. Immobilizing a 9-month-old infant.

Children should never be left unattended in a radiographic room for any reason. Many times, children are better behaved when their parents are not in the radiographic room. This is not always possible, especially when someone is needed to restrain the child. The best possible person to help restrain the patient is an older person. If the parents must be involved, follow the

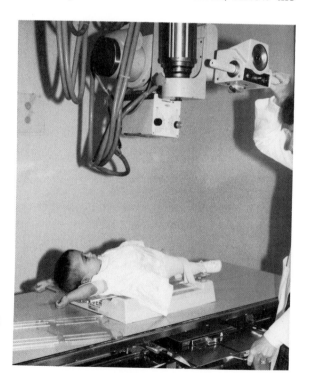

Fig. 11–3. Properly immobilized infant does not need to be held during radiographic examinations.

guidelines of your health facility. Make sure the restrainer is protected properly from scattered and secondary radiation by the use of lead rubber gloves and aprons. The collimation must keep the restrainer out of the area of the primary beam.

When taking radiographs of children, I recommend checking the first x-ray exposure for the proper technique. By following this simple rule, you take fewer repeat films, the x-radiation dose to the child is less, and you as the radiographer will feel better about the "case."

It takes patience and understanding to deal with children in a radiology department. If you are confident about the radiographic techniques that you use, it is a good bet that you will not shy away from pediatric radiography.

1. Osteoporosis is most common in:
   a. All women
   b. Oriental women
   c. Oriental men
   d. Caucasian women
   e. Caucasian women and men

2. The elderly usually have _____ pathologic conditions when compared with younger people.
   a. More
   b. Less
   c. The same number of

3. Pediatric patients have _____ percentage of water than geriatric patients.
   a. A higher
   b. A lower
   c. The same

4. Centimeter for centimeter, you should use _____ kVp for pediatric patients. Why?
   a. Higher
   b. Lower

5. Children are grouped into the 3- or 4-group classifications for radiographic technique until they reach about age _____ .

6. According to groupings by 4, figure the following techniques:
   a. Adult
      technique: 35 mAs
      80 kVp
      18-cm measurement
      Age 9 months: ? mAs
      ? kVp
      7-cm measurement
   b. Adult
      technique: 200 mA
      1/10 s
      66 kVp
      14-cm measurement
      Age 6 years: 400 mA
      ? s
      ? kVp
      8-cm measurement
   c. Adult
      technique: 300 mA
      50 ms
      95 kVp
      22-cm measurement
      Age 2 years: ? mA
      25 ms
      ? kVp
      11-cm measurement

7. According to groupings by 3, figure the following techniques:
   a. Adult
      technique: 40 mAs
      75 kVp
      16-cm measurement
      Age 27 months: ? mAs
      ? kVp
      6-cm measurement
   b. Adult
      technique: 400 mA
      25 ms
      88 kVp
      21-cm measurement
      Age 5 years: ? mAs
      ? kVp
      9-cm measurement

   c. Adult

      technique: 600 mA

             1/20 s

             92 kVp

             18-cm measurement

Age 10
years: 800 mA

       ? s

       ? kVp

       14-cm measurement

8. Why should a radiographer use a high mA station when radiographing children and the elderly?

9. Who is the best person to restrain a child being radiographed? Why?
   a. His 25-year-old mother
   b. The student radiographer
   c. A staff radiographer
   d. The child's 52-year-old grandmother

10. X-ray photons travel with more ease through _____ muscle tissue.
    a. Well-toned   b. Poor, weak

11. A rule of thumb to remember is to reduce the normal mAs by _____ % when radiographing the elderly.

12. Figure a radiographic technique for a patient who is 92 years old and is scheduled to have a radiographic examination of the pelvis. Normal adult technique is 22 mAs, 68 kVp for the measurement.

13. Discuss why the shoulder is an area of concern when radiographing the elderly.

12

Pathology and Radiographic Technique

OBJECTIVES *After completion of this chapter, the student radiographer should be able to:*

1. State the necessity of a clinical diagnosis for each patient that is radiographed.

2. Define pathologic conditions that are considered additive and those that are considered negative or destructive.

3. To figure new radiographic exposure techniques according to patient pathology.

4. To start to notice patient signs more carefully and to anticipate what radiographic technique changes are needed.

Clearly, not all patients fit into a "mold" that can be radiographed using certain factors so that all the films have the same type of density, contrast, and detail. Not only do we have patients with different tissue make-up, but also many patients that come to us have pathologic conditions. Pathology usually affects the radiographic density in one of two ways—*additive pathology* and *destructive pathology*. Additive pathology is a condition that requires the use of more mAs or more kVp. Destructive pathology has the opposite affect; the condition has destroyed some of the tissue and thus you must use less kVp or mAs. In either case, if the radiographer uses a technique for normal tissue, the result will not be what is needed for the proper image production. The image will be too dense or not dense enough.

Radiographers, of course, do not ask the patient for a diagnosis of his or her condition. Every patient that comes to the radiology department should have some type of clinical history available to the radiographer. Availability of this information is a great problem in many health facilities. If the request for a chest radiograph cites a clinical history of emphysema, the radiographer will realize that the radiographic technique must involve some type of compensation. In many cases, this information saves the patient from a repeat film.

There is no cut and dried way to deal with patient pathology from a radiographic standpoint. The amount of increase or decrease depends on the stage or progression of the patient's disease. We cannot, for instance, say that any patient suffering from emphysema needs 6 kVp less for a good film. One patient might have a mild form of emphysema whereas the next might have an advanced stage of the disease. I think the most important thing for the radiographer to realize is that they must use either more or less technique. Determining the actual degree of compensation becomes easier as you gain experience. What you must know is whether to add to the technique or subtract from it.

Many radiology departments post a list of pathologic conditions that require some compensation and the proper way to compensate. The following is a list of common pathologic conditions that are encountered in health facilities.

Additive Pathology
(Hard to penetrate)
Chest
   Aortic aneurysm
   Atelectasis
   Bronchiectasis
   Edema
   Empyema
   Enlarged heart
   Malignancy
   Pleural effusion
   Pneumonia

Skeletal system
   Acromegaly
   Exostosis
   Osteoma
   Paget's disease

Abdominal cavity
   Edema
   Cirrhosis

Destructive Pathology
(Easy to penetrate)
Chest
   Emphysema
   Pneumothorax
   Active tuberculosis

Skeletal system
   Active osteomyelitis
   Aseptic necrosis
   Atrophy
   Carcinoma
   Degenerative arthritis
   Gout
   Osteoporosis

Abdominal cavity
   Emaciation
   Pneumoperitoneum

You can see that this list only lets you know in what direction to change your technique.

The job of the radiographer is to be able to decide approximately how much to go up or down in technique. You must evaluate the condition of the patient from the standpoint of radiography. If the clinical history reads, "rule out a certain pathology," that does not necessarily mean that the patient has the disease, only that this radiographic procedure will act to rule out whether the patient actually has that disease.

As you go through your schooling, you will learn many of the telltale signs of some diseases, i.e., a patient suffering from emphysema might have a wheezing type of breathing or have a barrel-shaped chest from constantly gasping for enough oxygen and placing strain on the diaphragmatic muscle. As a first-year student, it is not easy to notice these signs. As you progress through your training, however, you will be able to correlate the clinical diagnosis with the patient signs and symptoms.

Normally, when you want to change a technique, you change either the kVp or the mAs. You know that a 30% change in the mAs produces a visible change in the overall density of a film. Therefore, if you need to compensate for some type of additive pathology and you want to use the mAs as the changeable factor, you should use an increase of at least 30%.

If you normally use a technique of 30 mAs for an abdominal radiographic image and the patient is suffering from cirrhosis, you should use 40 mAs:

$$\begin{array}{r} 30 \\ \times\ 0.30\ (\%) \\ \hline 9.0 \end{array}$$

The new mAs is 39, so use 40. This change should make a visible difference in the radiographic image.

If you decide to change the kVp, you must remember these two things: (1) The scale of contrast changes when you change the kVp, and (2) a 5% difference in kVp makes a visible difference in the radiographic image. If you are radiographing the abdomen of the patient suffering from cirrhosis and you normally use 30 mAs, 72 kVp for the radiographic technique of the normal patient, you should use at least 5% more kVp.

$$\begin{array}{r} 72 \\ \times\ 0.05 \\ \hline 3.60 \end{array}$$

Use 30 mAs, 76 kVp for the abdominal radiograph. Remember that 5% is 5%. It is *not* 6–8 kVp; 5% of 52 kVp is 3 kVp and 5% of 91 kVp is 5 kVp.

Your choice of method to use to increase the x-ray exposure (mAs amount or kVp penetration) makes a visible difference in the radiographic image. In some health facilities, you will be asked to increase the kVp and in others you will increase mAs. Many times, the radiographer is expected to make the decision.

ORTHOPEDIC CAST RADIOGRAPHY

At times, it is necessary to radiograph patients that have been immobilized with orthopedic casts. These devices are usually made of either plaster of paris (plaster cast) or fiberglass. These casts are radiographed when they are wet or dry. They present certain problems to the radiographer. A wet cast is more radiopaque than a dry cast. The general rule of thumb when radiographing patients wearing casts is as follows:

Wet plaster cast	3× normal mAs
Dry plaster cast	2× normal mAs
Wet fiberglass cast	Increase kVp by 5–6%
Dry fiberglass cast	No change is necessary

The kVp levels for patients with casts should be ascertained by measuring a comparable extremity. For example, if you must radiograph the left wrist with a cast, measure the right wrist. When a patient has bilateral casts, and many times they do because of multiple trauma, make a judgment call.

Let us work the following examples for cast technique. A patient has a dry plaster cast on his left knee because of a tibial plateau fracture. What technique should you use if the right knee measures 14 cm and the technique for a normal extremity is 5 mAs, 12:1 grid, 10 cm at 68 kVp?

Double the mAs. $2 \times 5 = 10$ mAs. If for 10 cm you use 68 kVp, add 2 kVp for each additional centimeter measurement. $4 \times 2 = 8$. $68 + 8 = 76$. If the plaster cast is wet (less than 24 hours old), you must use a multiple of 3. So the technique should be 15 mAs, 76 kVp.

A patient has a fiberglass cast on the wrist and the physician requests a postreduction radiograph. The cast was just applied; therefore, it is wet. What technique should you use?

The opposite wrist measures 4 cm. The normal radiographic technique for an upper extremity is 1.2 mAs, 6 cm, 58 kVp. For a noncasted 4-cm extremity, the kVp is 54. Add 5 to 6% more or 3 extra kVp. Use 1.2 mAs, 57 kVp.

1. Why is it important to have a clinical diagnosis on a radiographic requisition?

2. Destructive pathology necessitates a(an) _____ in x-ray penetration.
   a. Increase
   b. Decrease

3. A ____% increase or decrease in mAs makes a visible difference in the radiographic image.
   a. 5   b. 10   c. 20   d. 30   e. 40

4. A ____% increase or decrease in kVp makes a visible difference in the radiographic image.
   a. 5   b. 10   c. 15   d. 20   e. 30

5. A patient suffering from emphysema should have a(an) _____ in radiographic technique? Why?
   a. Increase
   b. Decrease

6. What are two clinical signs of a patient suffering from emphysema?

7. If you would use 77 kVp for a normal abdominal film, how much kVp should you use for a patient with cirrhosis of the liver?

8. If you would use 25 mAs for a normal lumbar spine radiograph, how much mAs should you use for a patient that has osteoporosis?

━ 13

Automatic Exposure Control Devices

OBJECTIVES *After completion of this chapter with the labs, the student radiographer should be able to:*

1. Define automatic exposure control devices and explain how they work.

2. Discuss the following with reference to automatic exposure control devices:
   a. Back-up exposure time
   b. kVp selection
   c. mA station selection
   d. Fields or chambers of automatic exposure control devices

3. State reasons when automatic exposure control devices should be used and when they should not be used.

Most modern radiographic equipment is equipped with automatic exposure control devices. In most radiography schools, these devices are used in conjunction with the clinical portion of the training. The use of these automatic exposure control devices sometimes has a negative effect on the student learning the principles of radiographic exposure. Unfortunately, many radiographers depend on the use of automatic exposure control devices, and when they are called on to work with manual techniques, they are unable to do so.

Automatic exposure control devices are a valuable asset to any radiology department. The use of these phototimers enables the department to produce radiographs with equal density regardless of the patients' pathologic condition. With the use of automatic exposure control devices, the radiographer does not have to make changes with regard to patient pathology.

RADIOGRAPHIC DENSITY

When using automatic exposure control devices, the exposure is terminated when the film in the cassette or holding apparatus receives a certain amount of x-radiation exposure. This amount is predetermined by how much density is selected. When this amount of exposure is reached, the x-ray exposure automatically shuts off.

The use of automatic exposure control devices does not eliminate the need for making choices by the radiographer. The radiographer must select the kVp for each exposure. In many health facilities, a particular kVp is used for each portion of the body, i.e., 80 kVp for skull radiography and 110 kVp for chest radiographs. Sometimes, the kVp selection is left up to the radiographer. If you are given this option to choose for yourself, it is important to remember two things: (1) When you select relatively high kVp, the patient receives less x-radiation. (2) If you do not use a kVp that is able to penetrate the subject, the radiographic image will not have enough density (regardless of the mAs used). Always use more than the minimum kVp required for any body part. If the kVp is higher than normal, however, the radiographic image will have a scale of contrast that is too long and the film will be too gray and "washed out." With most automatic exposure control devices, the radiographer selects all the radiographic factors with the exception of the exposure time. With most machines, a back-up time is used. This is a safety device in case the machine malfunctions.

When selecting mA station, it is important to use one that is reasonable. Avoid excessively high settings because of response time and also because if a malfunction occurs and the exposure uses all the back-up time, the patient receives more radiation. For example, if the back-up time is 1 second, use of an 800 mA station allows 800 mAs.* If back-up time is 1 second and the 300 mA station is selected, only 300 mAs is delivered if the machine malfunctions.

You also must be careful not to use an mA setting that is too low. If you choose the 25 mA setting with a back-up time of 1 second, you cannot use more than 25 mAs for any single exposure. If an abdominal film requires 35 mAs and the settings only allow you to use 25 mAs, the film will not have enough density. Most companies recommend using mA stations from about 200 to 600 when using automatic exposure control devices.

IONIZATION CHAMBERS AND PHOTO CELLS

The most accurate type of automatic exposure control device is the ionization chamber. They are radiolucent and must be situated between the patient and the film.

Some machines have only one chamber or photocell located in the center of the area to be radiographed (Fig. 13–1). More sophisticated machines have three or four fields or chambers (Fig. 13–2). The radiographer has the option of using only the center field, any other chamber, or even all three or four chambers. Whatever way the chambers are selected, the exposure will not be terminated until all the chambers selected have received enough radiation to allow for the predetermined radiographic density. The radiographer must strive to select the correct chamber. If the wrong field is selected, it might mean the film must be repeated. For example, if the radiographer selects the center field for a posteroanterior projection of the chest, the ionization chamber would not shut off the exposure until the area including the mediastinum has suf-

---

*The Department of Health and Human Services states that no phototimed exposure shall exceed a total of 800 mAs. The x-ray machines must be equipped with some type of circuit breaker that will not allow any mAs of greater than 800 in case of machine malfunction.

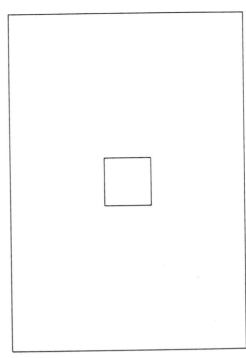

Fig. 13–1. Automatic exposure control device, single field.

ficient density; by that time, the lungs appear almost black on the radiographic film.

Another important consideration when working with automatic exposure control devices is the centering of the part to the field. If you are radiographing the lumbar spine in the lateral projection, be sure that the spine is centered

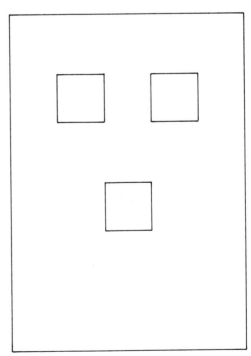

Fig. 13–2. Automatic exposure control device, multiple fields.

on the film. If for some reason the spine is located on either side of center, the exposure will shut off before the spine area has received enough x-radiation. This centering is often a problem when radiographing the cervical spine in the erect lateral projection, especially if the patient has a tendency to sway.

In many radiology departments, radiographers use automatic exposure control devices for barium radiographic studies. Most of the time, no problems arise with this procedure. Sometimes, however, when using the center field and radiographing the stomach that is filled with barium, the exposure lasts too long, causing the film to have too much density. The reason for this increased density is that the chamber is right under the filled stomach and this area does not receive enough x-radiation to satisfy the requirements of the film density. When you view the image, the surrounding, overexposed area is black and the center of the stomach is still clear. For this reason, it is important not to use a back-up that increases the radiation dose to the patient: Suppose you use a back-up time of 0.5s and mA of 200. The most exposure the patient could receive is 100 mAs. If you use a back-up time of 1.5s and mA of 400, the patient could receive 600 mAs if the chamber is under a large, filled stomach.

The same type of situation could happen when performing barium enemas and double-contrast barium enemas. You could produce a light film if the chamber is located just under a bowel segment filled only with air (negative contrast). Because of these problems, I do not recommend the use of automatic exposure control devices for gastrointestinal radiographic examinations.

1. Automatic exposure control devices used in a radiology department allow radiographers to keep _____ equal on all patients.
   a. Contrast
   b. Density
   c. Distortion
   d. Patient dose

2. The radiographer can choose any kVp that he or she wants when working with automatic exposure control devices.
   (   ) True   (   ) False

3. What problems might be encountered when choosing kVp that is _____?
   Explain each.
   a. Relatively low   b. Relatively high

4. Department of Health and Human Services regulations state that no phototimed exposure can exceed a potential of _____ mAs.
   a. 200   b. 400   c. 600   d. 800

5. The most accurate type of automatic exposure control device is the
   _____.

6. Which photocell(s) should be activated when radiographing the chest in the posteroanterior position?
   1. Center field   2. Lateral fields   3. All fields
   a. All the above   c. 2 only
   b. 1 only   d. Any of the above

7. When radiographing the lumbar spine in the lateral position and the abdomen instead of the spine is located above the photocell, the radiograph would probably demonstrate:
   a. Sufficient density at the lumbar area
   b. Insufficient density at the lumbar area
   c. Too much density at the lumbar area
   d. A scale of contrast that is too long

8. What might be the probable cause of a lack of density in barium enema air contrast radiograph taken in conjunction with an automatic exposure control device?

LAB No. 1

Necessary Equipment

1. Energized x-ray room with automatic exposure control device with multiple fields
2. Processor
3. 14 × 17-inch cassette filled
4. Chest phantom

Expose the phantom in the posteroanterior or anteroposterior position using the center field cell for one exposure and the lateral field cells for a second exposure. Compare the processed films. Notice that the first film has too much density.

LAB No. 2

Necessary Equipment

1. Energized x-ray room with automatic exposure control device with multiple fields.
2. Processor
3. 14 × 17-inch cassette filled
4. Abdomen phantom

Place the phantom in the center of the table. Expose the lateral lumbar area using the center field cells. Take a second exposure, but move the phantom so the spine is no longer centered. Again, expose the film using the center field cell. Check the processed films. Notice that the second film demonstrates insufficient density over the lumbar area.

14

Preparing Radiographic Technique Charts

OBJECTIVES *After completion of this chapter with the labs, the student radiographer should be able to:*

1. List the reasons for radiographic technique changes in normal charts.

2. List radiographic equipment necessary for formulating radiographic technique charts.

3. Define the two types of radiographic technique charts.

4. Figure radiographic exposure techniques for the variable kVp techniques chart and the fixed kVp techniques chart.

Some ground rules must be considered before attempting to create a radiographic technique chart. Even after you have learned the material in the previous chapters, many more little truisms that pertain to radiography remain. The following is a list to consider:

1. When radiographing the abdomen with the added factor of barium, you must double the technique: use 2 times mAs *or* 15% more kVp.
2. A lateral projection of the chest usually requires using twice as much mAs as is used for a posteroanterior projection.
3. For the anteroposterior projection of the ankle, use 2 kVp more than the measurement suggests.
4. An RAO (right anterior oblique) view of the esophagus requires using one half the technique used for a similar projection of the stomach.
5. For a lateral film of the lumbar spine, use 2 times the mAs technique you use for an anteroposterior view of this region.
6. You should not use more than 85 kVp when the contrast medium is iodine. The addition of iodine as the contrast agent requires the use of about 4 kVp higher than normal.
7. When changing from a posteroanterior or anteroposterior position of the abdomen to a 45° oblique, you need about 6 to 8 more kVp.

Before any person begins to formulate a radiographic technique chart, they must know a few things about the radiology department and the machines that they will use. These considerations are as follows:

1. Type of grids in tables, types of grids for portables.
2. Type of x-ray generation (single phase or three phase).
3. Type of film/screen combination.
4. Type of film density the radiologists require for the radiographs.
5. Type of film contrast the radiologists require for the radiographs.
6. How much collimation is used for various examinations.
7. The focal-film distances (FFD) used.

Two types of radiographic technique charts that can be employed: The variable kVp chart and the fixed kVp (variable mAs) chart.

VARIABLE kVp TECHNIQUE CHART

The variable kVp chart was the first type used in radiology departments. Use of early charts of this type usually resulted in high radiation doses to the patient because most often they utilized minimal kVp. I do not think this is the proper way to formulate such a chart. I advocate the use of relatively high kVp. Early charts usually used the rule of thumb to determine the kVp (2 × cm + 25 or 30). I suggest a kVp setting of about 20 to 25 kVp higher than the minimum for imaging the extremities and about 10 to 20 kVp higher for other body areas. A higher setting allows for lower mAs settings.

When you begin a variable kVp technique, a caliper is important, as is the way it is used. You must have accurate measurements of the anatomic parts or the kVp will be either too low or too high. Variable kVp charts (Figs. 14–1 and 14–2) use a sliding kVp of 2 for each centimeter of thickness after the standard is set. If you use 60 kVp for a 6-cm thickness, you should use 62 for 7 cm, 58 for 5 cm, and so on. Once you have figured the technique for certain body parts, the rest is easy.

Suppose you must figure a technique for the following:

1. An extremity
2. The skull
3. The abdomen
4. Chest

To start the chart, you must have radiographic phantoms (Fig. 14–3). For the extremity technique, select the phantom and measure it properly. Let us say you selected a hand phantom that measures 4 cm for the posteroanterior projection. Minimum kVp would be 33 or 38. To start, I would use a kVp setting of 52 to 56. (Remember that higher kVp is better for the patient.) Select the kVp and take exposures starting at mAs settings that you consider too low. This setting depends mainly on the film/screen combination you are using. Increase the mAs for subsequent exposures by about 30%. Make sure the FFD is accurately set at the desired level. Use the amount of collimation that you will use consistently. Place the finished radiographs on identical viewboxes and check the results. Compare the radiographs and determine which has the proper amount of density. After this process is complete, you have the tech-

CHEST

POSITION	MA	SEC	DIST	CM	14	16	18	20	22	24	26	28	30	32	34	36	38	40	42
PA				K															
LAT				V															
OBL																			
APICAL																			

ESOPHAGUS

POSITION	MA	SEC	DIST	CM	14	16	18	20	22	24	26	28	30	32	34	36	38	40	42
PA				K															
LAT				V															
L. OBL.																			
R. OBL.																			

RIBS (ABOVE DIAPHRAGM)

POSITION	MA	SEC	DIST	CM	14	16	18	20	22	24	26	28	30	32	34	36	38	40	42
AP or PA				K															
OBL				V															

RIBS (BELOW DIAPHRAGM)

POSITION	MA	SEC	DIST	CM	12	14	16	18	20	22	24	26	28	30	32	34	36	38	40
AP or PA				K															
OBL				V															

ABDOMEN—K.U.B.

POSITION	MA	SEC	DIST	CM	12	14	16	18	20	22	24	26	28	30	32	34	36	38	40
AP or PA				K															
LAT. DEC.				V															
ERECT																			
OBL																			

G. I. SERIES

POSITION	MA	SEC	DIST	CM	12	14	16	18	20	22	24	26	28	30	32	34	36	38	40
PA				K															
1st OBL				V															
2nd OBL																			
LAT																			

BA. ENEMA

POSITION	MA	SEC	DIST	CM	12	14	16	18	20	22	24	26	28	30	32	34	36	38	40
AP or PA				K															
OBL				V															
LAT. RECT.																			
POST. EVAC																			
ANG. SIG.																			

BA. ENEMA (AIR CONT).

POSITION	MA	SEC	DIST	CM	12	14	16	18	20	22	24	26	28	30	32	34	36	38	40
AP or PA				K															
OBL				V															
LAT																			

GALL BLADDER

POSITION	MA	SEC	DIST	CM	12	14	16	18	20	22	24	26	28	30	32	34	36	38	40
PA				K															
OBL				V															
ERECT																			
LAT. DEC.																			

Fig. 14–1. Variable kVp technique chart. (Courtesy of Fuji Medical Systems U.S.A., Inc.) *Continued on following pages.*

SKULL

POSITION	MA	SEC	DIST	CM	12	13	14	15	16	17	18	19	20	21	22	23	24	25	26	27
TOWNE'S				K																
AP or PA				V																
LAT																				
BASAL																				

SINUSES

POSITION	MA	SEC	DIST	CM	12	13	14	15	16	17	18	19	20	21	22	23	24	25	26	27
CALDWELL				K																
WATER'S				V																
LAT																				
BASAL																				
ETHMOID																				

MASTOIDS

POSITION	MA	SEC	DIST	CM	12	13	14	15	16	17	18	19	20	21	22	23	24	25	26	27
TOWNE'S				K																
LAW'S				V																
STENVER'S																				
SCHULER'S																				
TIPS																				

MANDIBLE & TMJ's

POSITION	MA	SEC	DIST	CM	8	9	10	11	12	13	14	15	16	17	18	19	20	21	22	23
PA or AP				K																
OBL				V																
T.M.J. LAT.																				

NASAL BONES

POSITION	MA	SEC	DIST	CM	12	13	14	15	16	17	18	19	20	21	22	23	24	25	26	27
SCREEN/CARD				K																
WATER'S				V																
PA or AP																				
SUPERO-INF																				

CERVICAL SPINE

POSITION	MA	SEC	DIST	CM	7	8	9	10	11	12	13	14	15	16	17	18	19	20	21	22
AP				K																
LAT				V																
OBL																				
ODONTOID.																				

THORACIC SPINE

POSITION	MA	SEC	DIST	CM	14	16	18	20	22	24	26	28	30	32	34	36	38	40	42	44
AP				K																
LAT				V																
OBL																				

LUMBAR SPINE

POSITION	MA	SEC	DIST	CM	12	14	16	18	20	22	24	26	28	30	32	34	36	38	40	42
AP or PA				K																
LAT				V																
L5-S1																				
OBL																				

SACRUM

POSITION	MA	SEC	DIST	CM	12	14	16	18	20	22	24	26	28	30	32	34	36	38	40	42
AP				K																
LAT				V																

COCCYX

POSITION	MA	SEC	DIST	CM	12	14	16	18	20	22	24	26	28	30	32	34	36	38	40	42
AP				K																
LAT				V																

Fig. 14–1. *Continued.*

SHOULDER

POSITION	MA	SEC	DIST	CM	10	12	14	16	18	20	22	24	26	28	30	32	34	36	38	40
AP				K																
AP (Int.Rot.)				V																
AP (Ext.Rot.)																				
TRA/THOR																				

SCAPULA

POSITION	MA	SEC	DIST	CM	10	12	14	16	18	20	22	24	26	28	30	32	34	36	38	40
AP				K																
LAT				V																

CLAVICLE

POSITION	MA	SEC	DIST	CM	10	12	14	16	18	20	22	24	26	28	30	32	34	36	38	40
AP or PA				K																
INFERO-SUP.				V																

ACROMIO-CLAV.JTS.

POSITION	MA	SEC	DIST	CM	10	12	14	16	18	20	22	24	26	28	30	32	34	36	38	40
AP																				

STERNUM & S.C.JTS.

POSITION	MA	SEC	DIST	CM	12	14	16	18	20	22	24	26	28	30	32	34	36	38	40	42
PA				K																
OBL (Breathing)				V																
OBL (Arrested)																				

PELVIS

POSITION	MA	SEC	DIST	CM	14	16	18	20	22	24	26	28	30	32	34	36	38	40	42	44
AP				K																
OBL				V																
LAT																				

HIP

POSITION	MA	SEC	DIST	CM	12	14	16	18	20	22	24	26	28	30	32	34	36	38	40	42
AP				K																
LAT				V																

FEMUR

POSITION	MA	SEC	DIST	CM	6	7	8	9	10	11	12	13	14	15	16	17	18	19	20	21
AP				K																
LAT				V																

KNEE

POSITION	MA	SEC	DIST	CM	6	7	8	9	10	11	12	13	14	15	16	17	18	19	20	21
AP				K																
LAT				V																
OBL																				
TANGENTIAL																				
TUNNEL																				

PELVIMETRY

POSITION	MA	SEC	DIST	CM	16	18	20	22	24	26	28	30	32	34	36	38	40	42	44	46
AP				K																
LAT				V																
LAT (Placenta)																				
THOMS																				
ERECT																				

EXTREMITIES

TECHNIQUE	MA	SEC	DIST	CM	1	2	3	4	5	6	7	8	9	10	11	12	13	14	15	16
NON-SCREEN				K																
SCREEN				V																

Fig. 14–1. *Continued.*

nique for nonBucky imaging of the extremities. Fill in the kVp levels for the different centimeter thicknesses.

Exposure	kVp	mAs
1	54	1
2	54	1.3
3	54	1.7
4	54	2.2
5	54	2.8

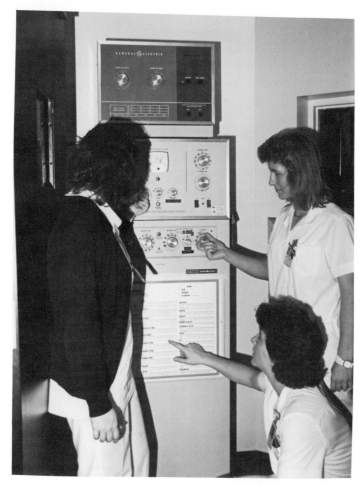

Fig. 14–2. Radiography students consulting a technique chart for proper radiographic factors.

This chart should work well for all "non-pathology" studies of the extremities. Remember to make a note that the anteroposterior projection of the ankle should be taken with a kVp that is equal to the norm for the patient measurement plus 2.

For patients with certain pathologic conditions (categories discussed in Chapter 12), you should figure the proper compensation in technique before the first x-ray exposure. As an example, for a patient with severe osteoarthritis, use less kVp than the patient measurement suggests. This same chart can be used if you decide to use the Bucky grid for the exposures. Just multiply the mAs by the proper factor for the grid, i.e., when using 1.3 mAs for a non-Bucky technique and the table is equipped with a 12:1 grid, the proper mAs is 6.5, with the kVp for the patient measurement.

As a working radiographer, it is not necessary to measure a wrist three times or an ankle three times to set the proper kVp levels. Once you measure the wrist in the posteroanterior position, just add 2 kVp for the oblique view and another 2 kVp for the lateral view. When measuring the ankle, the opposite occurs. If you measure the ankle in the anteroposterior position to determine

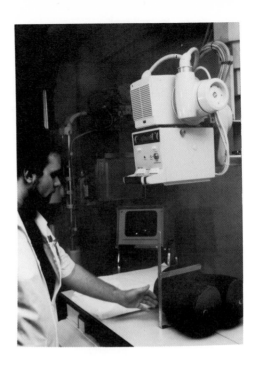

Fig. 14–3. Radiographer preparing for radiographic technique chart.

starting kVp levels (which are 2 kVp more than normal measurement), use 2 kVp less than the anteroposterior measurement for the oblique view and another 2 kVp less for the lateral view. With instruction regarding extremity positioning, you can determine what views need more and what views need less kVp than the original measurement. At certain times, you might want to perform more measurements for the same area; for example when you must radiograph a patient with some type of extremity deformity or when the amount of obliquity is different than normal.

Next, prepare a technique for the skull. The normal lateral skull measured between the parietal eminences (the widest portion of a lateral skull) is 14 cm. The normal Caldwell measurement is 19 cm (central ray travels from the upper parietal area to the nasion). You do not need the large sliding kVp ranges that are necessary for extremities.

	kVp										
	12	13	14	15	16	17	18	19	20	21	22
Lateral		66	68	70							
Caldwell posteroanterior projection						74	76	78	80	82	
Grashey anteroposterior axial projection							76	78	80	82	84
Schuller full base								78	80	82	84

Place the skull phantom in the lateral position and select a kVp. Select the mAs that you think is low and expose the films, increasing the mAs by about 30% for each film. Once again, evaluate the radiographs and decide on the proper density. If you want to try another kVp, by all means do so. By changing the kVp, of course, the radiographic contrast also changes. Only by this trial and error method will you arrive at the contrast that the radiologist needs to make a proper interpretation of the radiographs. You may decide that a change in mAs is necessary for the other skull films. If so, the kVp levels may change also. After the routine skull views are perfected, you can continue with the more advanced skull areas, such as the facial bones, the mastoids, and so on.

Working on the techniques for the abdomen are probably the most time-consuming. After you follow the procedure to determine the radiographic technique for the abdomen, you can then convert this technique to the other areas within the abdominal cavity. Let us say that you established a technique of 20 mAs, 78 kVp for a patient who has a measurement of 19 cm. You are now able to make techniques for other areas. Let us work a few examples.

PROBLEM 1: Intravenous pyelogram, 14 × 17-inch anteroposterior film. The patient measurement is 16 cm. Use 20 mAs at 76 kVp. Normally, you use 72 kVp for a 16 cm. When iodine is used as the contrast material, you add 4 kVp.

If the kVp is higher than 82, you must then use more mAs so you can lower the kVp.

For the same study, you are to use 20 mAs, 88 kVp and the patient measurement is 22 cm. This kVp is too high to be used with iodine as a contrast medium. Simply increase the mAs by 2 times and reduce the kVp by 15%. The new technique is 40 mAs, 75 kVp.

PROBLEM 2: Barium enema, 14 × 17-inch anteroposterior film, double technique. The patient measurement is 18 cm. Use (A) 20 mAs, 86 kVp or (B) 10 mAs, 99 kVp. For A, the technique was doubled by adding 15% to the kVp. For B, you do the same thing as in A but you carry it one step further. Divide the mAs by 2 and add 15% kVp. Both A and B have equal density.

PROBLEM 3: Anteroposterior view of the lumbar spine. The patient measurement is 22 cm. The normal technique for a 22-cm measurement is 20 mAs, 84 kVp. What you must remember is that the collimation should be reduced to about 7 × 17 inches so the mAs is increased to compensate for the lessening of the scattered and secondary radiation reaching the film. A 7 × 17-inch field size is equal to a 10 × 12-inch film (7 × 17 = 119 and 10 × 12 = 120). Therefore, you must use about 20% more mAs. The new technique is 24 to 25 mAs, 84 kVp. If you want or need a shorter scale of contrast, reduce the kVp by 15% (84 − 15% [12.6 or 13] = 71 kVp) and double the mAs (24 to 25 × 2 = 48 or 50). Note: When changing the lumbar spine technique from the anteroposterior to the lateral position, double the mAs and the kVp should reflect the lateral measurement.

PROBLEM 4: Stomach filled with barium, 10 × 12-inch, right anterior oblique position. The patient measurement is 19 cm. Double the technique with the addition of barium, 20 mAs, 88 kVp. Add 6 kVp for the oblique view, 20 mAs, 94 kVp. Add 20% mAs because of film size. New technique is 24 to 25 mAs, 94 kVp, which will produce a film with density equal to that in the abdominal film.

You can see that we could go on and on with these problems. If a technique chart is posted in the radiology department, simply measure the patient and set the technique accordingly. If the technique is set up properly, the kVp will reflect the addition of barium, air, or iodine as the contrast material. When the kVp is too high for iodine use, compensate by decreasing the kVp and increasing the mAs accordingly. You should see an increase in kVp but not the mAs when working with barium. Some departments use a standard kVp for barium studies and others use a range of kVp.

Once you get started on the technique chart, it is not difficult to continue until all anatomic areas are finished.

To make a chest technique chart, use a chest phantom. Decide whether to use a grid and, if so, what grid ratio. Place the chest phantom against the wall film holder in the posteroanterior position. Make radiographic exposures, starting with proper kVp and using a mAs setting that you consider slightly inadequate. Make an additional exposure, increasing the mAs by about 30%. Compare the radiographs and determine which has the proper density. After the proper radiographic technique is determined for this projection, turn the phantom to the lateral position. Measure for the proper kVp setting and use 2 times the mAs used for the posteroanterior projection. Make additional exposures, using 30% more mAs and 30% less mAs to make sure that the proper density is selected.

FIXED kVp TECHNIQUE CHART

In many health facilities, radiographers use the fixed kVp technique chart. Many experts think the patient dose of x-radiation is less with this method. I do not share this belief because I recommend relatively high kVp for my variable kVp charts. When preparing fixed kVp charts, the first step is to determine what kVp to use for each body part. Let us say you choose to use 80 kVp for a radiograph of the abdomen. Start with an mAs setting that you consider insufficient and take the first film. Take additional films, with 30 to 35% more mAs, until you find the proper density. For all of these films, use a phantom of medium size (22 cm). The next step is to divide the abdomen into three major groups, small: 12–18, medium: 19–24, and large: 25–30. Use the technique for the medium abdomen for normal patients that measure between 19 and 24 cm. For the small patient, use about 30% less mAs; for the large patient, use about 30% more mAs. I find many times that when following these charts, radiographs taken of the patients at the ends of the scale are either lacking in density or possess too much density.

Some experts say that all films taken at a particular kVp have the same contrast. In actual practice, however, this statement is not true. When using 80 kVp to image an anatomic part that measures 15 cm and the same kVp on one that measures 20 cm, the amount of attenuation of the x-ray photons is not the same. The subject contrast alters the scale of contrast on the radiograph. With this type of chart, you also must adjust the kVp when the patient is larger than the size for which you use minimum kVp levels (2 × cm + 25 or 30).

A newer type of technique chart is the high kVp technique chart. These charts are becoming more popular because of the extremely long scale of contrast produced on the radiographs. They also incorporate minimal mAs, a practice that is good for lowering the patient dose of x-radiation.

According to the National Council on Radiation Protection, all radiography rooms should be used in conjunction with a technique chart. No matter which type of chart you use, remember these charts are for radiographers, not button pushers. If the chart calls for 50 mAs, *you* have the choice as to how to arrive at the 50 mAs—maybe 500 mA and 1/10 s or 250 mA and 1/5 s. If you are radiographing a patient who is unable to hold his or her breath, you might want to use 1000 mA and 1/20 s. Remember, too, to change the factors for patients with pathologic conditions that warrant adjustment.

So you see, radiology technique charts are not put up for the department dummies, but rather to enhance the quality of the radiographs produced and to limit the number of repeated films.

1. How should an abdomen radiographic technique be altered for a barium enema?
   1. Add 10 kVp
   2. Increase the technique by 15% mAs
   3. Increase the technique by 15% kVp
   a. Any one of the above   c. 2 only
   b. 2 and 3   d. 3 only

2. A lateral chest radiograph usually requires using _____ mAs as for the posteroanterior projection.
   a. 2 times   c. Equal
   b. 3 times   d. One half the

3. The upper limits of kVp to use in conjunction with iodine as a contrast medium for radiography is _____.
   a. 60   b. 75   c. 80   d. 85

4. When changing from a posteroanterior or anteroposterior position for an intravenous pyelogram to an oblique view, the technique change should be:
   a. Add 6 to 8 kVp   c. Double the mAs
   b. Subtract 6 to 8 kVp   d. Use one half the mAs

5. What are the two most common radiographic technique charts used in radiology departments?
   1.
   2.

6. What is the rule of thumb to figure minimum kVp levels in radiography?

7. The usual difference in kVp for each centimeter of patient thickness is:
   a. 1   b. 2   c. 3   d. 4

8. What should be the difference between an anteroposterior abdomen technique and an anteroposterior lumbar spine technique?
   a. No difference   c. 20% less mAs
   b. 20% more mAs   d. 15% more kVp
   e. 15% less kVp

9. When figuring a technique that uses about 30% more mAs for a large abdominal radiograph than it does for a normal-sized abdominal film, you are working with a _____ type of radiographic chart.

10. High kVp techniques are useful for chest radiography. Why?

LAB No. 1

Necessary Equipment

1. Energized x-ray room
2. Skull or abdominal phantom
3. 14 × 17- or 10 × 12-inch cassettes filled
4. Film processor

Figure a variable kVp technique for either a lateral view of the skull or an anteroposterior view of the abdomen using the method discussed in this chapter. This lab will probably be more beneficial if you use a different than normal grid in the radiographic table or if you use a different film/screen combination than is normally used. You have an advantage if you leave everything the same because most students have an idea of proper technique for a particular radiographic room.

LAB No. 2

Using the same equipment, prepare a fixed kVp technique for either the skull or the abdominal phantom. Again, try to use other than normal accessories for this lab.

LAB No. 3

Necessary Equipment

1. Energized x-ray room
2. Film processor
3. Chest phantom
4. 14 × 17-inch cassettes
5. Rad check or dosimeter

Check with your clinical instructor as to the feasibility of this experiment in your radiology department.

Starting technique for posteroanterior projection of the chest:

1. 110 kVp
2. 72-inch FFD
3. Grid or nongrid, depending on facility
4. Start with low mAs, i.e., 1.5 with 8:1 grid, 0.375 nongrid.

Check this test film. Depending on the density, take subsequent films, increasing or decreasing the mAs by about 30% for each film. Compare the films to determine the proper film density for your radiology department.

■— *15*

Radiographic Tube Rating and Cooling Charts

OBJECTIVES *After completion of this chapter, the student radiographer should be able to:*

1. Identify the x-ray tube rating charts and be able to figure safe exposures for x-ray tubes.

2. Figure heat units for various x-ray techniques.

3. Differentiate between radiographic techniques that are safe and unsafe for the tubes.

4. Discuss how tube heat is dissipated from x-ray tubes.

5. Operate x-ray tubes according to safe limits.

6. Determine when excessive heat might be applied to the x-ray tube.

7. Allow for the proper cooling time between x-ray exposures or series of exposures.

The radiographic tube is an expensive piece of equipment that is under the almost direct influence of the radiographer. The life expectancy of a tube can be attributed directly to its use or misuse. A general purpose diagnostic tube can last 10 years or more if it is treated with care. The price of x-ray tubes used in general diagnostic radiography is in a range of $6,000.00 to $10,000.00 per tube. Larger and more sophisticated tubes used for serial radiography and computed tomography can cost as much as $36,000.00 per tube. You can see that if you obtain a job as a radiographer and the tube you use must be replaced every year or so, you are not much of an asset to your employer. Each and every x-ray tube sold comes with a minimum of three types of charts to be used in conjunction with that particular tube. They are the following:

1. Tube rating chart (one for each filament size)
2. Anode cooling chart
3. Tube housing cooling chart

Before you can understand how to operate these charts, you must be able to understand the thermal capacity of x-ray tubes. This thermal energy is converted to *heat units* (HU). The amount of heat units applied to the tubes depends on the radiographic technique employed. If you have studied x-ray generation, you realize that three-phase equipment generates more heat than single-phase x-ray equipment. The following are the formulas to use to determine heat units produced by a particular x-ray exposure or series of exposures:

$$\text{Single phase: Heat units} = \text{mA} \times \text{s} \times \text{kVp}$$

$$\text{Three phase: Heat units} = \text{mA} \times \text{s} \times \text{kVp} \times 1.35^*$$

If your technique is 300 mA, 1/10 s, 80 kVp using single-phase equipment, figure $300 \times 1/10 \times 80 = 2400$ HU. The same technique using three-phase equipment is $300 \times 1/10 \times 80 \times 1.35 = 3240$ HU.

When it is desirable to reduce the number of heat units, use a longer scale of contrast. Using the preceding example with single-phase equipment:

$$30 \text{ mAs} \times 80 \text{ kVp} = 2400 \text{ HU}$$

$$15 \text{ mAs} \times 92 \text{ kVp} = 1380 \text{ HU}$$

$$7.5 \text{ mAs} \times 106 \text{ kVp} = 795 \text{ HU}$$

Look what happens if the contrast is increased or shortened:

$$60 \text{ mAs} \times 68 \text{ kVp} = 4080 \text{ HU}$$

As a student radiographer, you know that about 99.8% of the energy needed to produce x-rays is converted into heat. It is this massive amount of heat that has the most detrimental effect on the x-ray tubes; it has the ability to melt or crack the tube anode. It is important that x-ray tubes are constructed so that heat dissipation is accomplished in the quickest and most effective manner. This heat is dissipated through the anode assembly. Most anodes today are constructed of *tungsten* coated with *rhenium.* The melting point of tungsten is about 3333° C. Rhenium is used to prevent the tungsten from pitting. Directly behind the stem is a copper shank that effectively removes heat. Some anodes are produced with a larger face; some also have graphite on the back side of the anode. Many anodes are equipped with stress-relieved construction. Radiography tubes are manufactured with rotating anodes that rotate either at low speed (3600 rpm) or at high speed 10,000 rpm). Because of this rotation, all heat produced by an exposure is not applied to one small area of the target. By this method, the heat is applied equally to the entire anode. When this heat is distributed equally, it is easier to dissipate.

Most x-ray tubes are manufactured with two filaments. The smaller should be used when detail is important and the larger should be used in conjunction with large or heavy exposures. The radiographer who uses the small filament constantly is not following good radiographic technique. A good radiographer considers all radiographic factors involved before selecting a technique. (This

---

*Some authorities use mA × s × kVp × 1.41

consideration must include not only patient factors but also x-ray tube features.) The profit margin is reduced severely if too many x-ray tubes must be purchased each year. Therefore, be sure that you use the tubes properly and that you understand how to interpret the safety charts for each tube.

TUBE RATING

These charts inform the radiographer as to how much kVp, mA, and time can be used safely for each filament of the tube (Fig. 15–1).

You probably cannot overload a properly functioning x-ray tube with one single heavy exposure because of the installation of appropriate circuit breakers. The machine will not make the exposure if too much kVp, mA, or time is selected. A print-out may appear on the console that reads "technique overload." The purpose of tube rating charts is so that you do not use techniques that are just under the tube overload. You should not use the tube for exposures that are close to the maximum. When you do approach the maximum, you shorten the life expectancy of that tube, especially when working with tomographic examinations or serial radiography.

You can see by studying Figures 15–1 and 15–2 that you can use either the mA station or the kVp as a variable. It depends on the manufacturer. By using these charts properly, you can keep the x-ray exposures below the maximum.

For example, you want to use (Fig. 15–1) a technique of 0.01 s, 120 kVp, 1200 mA. Find 0.01 on the chart and find 120 kVp on the chart. Notice that they meet above the 1200 mA line; therefore, this exposure cannot be applied safely to this tube. You could safely use any mA station below 1000 with 120 kVp and 0.01 s, but not 1200 or 1250. What is the maximum kVp you could use at 0.5-second exposure time using the 800 mA station? Locate 0.5 and

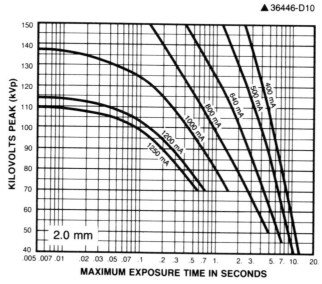

▲ 36446-D10

Fig. 15–1. Tube rating chart with mA used as the variable. (Courtesy of General Electric Company, Medical Systems Group, Milwaukee, WI.)

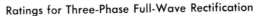

Ratings for Three-Phase Full-Wave Rectification

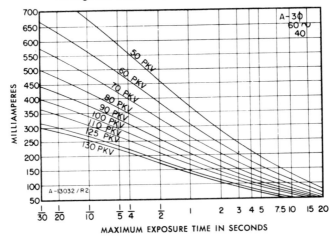

Fig. 15–2. Tube rating chart with kVp used as the variable. (Courtesy of Machlett Laboratories Inc., Springdale, CT.)

follow up to 800 mA, look to the left, and see that you could safely use just slightly above 90 kVp.

Now use the chart in Figure 15–2 and see if you can safely use 1/5 s, 400 mA, 80 kVp. Locate 1/5 at the bottom and follow this up to the 400 mA station. Notice that you cannot use 80 kVp safely. You could use 1/5 s, 200 mA, 92 kVp with no trouble (equal density film). Do you see how previous knowledge can help you? What is the highest kVp you could use safely with this chart, using 1-second exposure time and the 300 mA station? Answer: Just over 60.

When you check the tube rating charts in the radiography rooms, the charts for the large focal spot allow you to use heavier x-ray exposures. Why? Because you are using a larger area of the target at any given time. Realize, however, that when using the larger focal spot size, more geometric unsharpness is evident on the radiographic film image. As the tube ages, the target becomes more crazed and pitted. This crazing and pitting actually increases the size of the focal spot because of the tiny hills and valleys on the target. These tube rating charts are probably the most important charts used in general diagnostic radiography to prolong the life of the tube.

ANODE COOLING

Each anode has the capacity to store just so much heat before damage is rendered to that tube. Again, this heat is measured in heat units. Even though this tube is continually dissipating this heat, it is possible to apply too much (especially with serial exposures and/or tomographic exposures).

Figure 15–3 represents a typical anode cooling chart. You can see that you are able to put 140,000 HU on the anode before you reach the maximum. The actual amount of heat that can be applied is greater, because as soon as any exposure is finished, the anode begins to dissipate the heat. These charts are

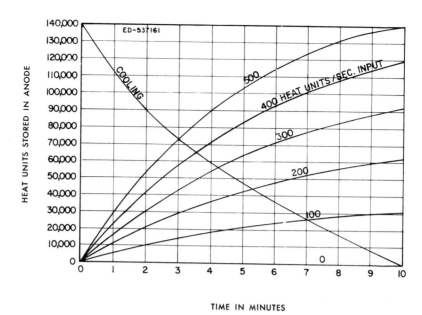

Fig. 15–3. Anode cooling chart. (Courtesy of Machlett Laboratories Inc., Springdale, CT.)

useful when taking serial films. Suppose the following technique is used for an aorta study in special procedures:

50 mAs
85 kVp
Three-phase rectification
Series: 4 films per second for 4 seconds
       3 films per second for 3 seconds
       2 films per second for 4 seconds

To work this problem, apply the formula to determine heat units:

$$50 \text{ mAs} \times 85 \text{ kVp} \times 1.35 = 5737.5 \text{ HU each exposure}$$

$$
\begin{aligned}
\text{Total exposures: } 4 \times 4 &= 16 \\
3 \times 3 &= 9 \\
2 \times 4 &= \underline{8} \\
&\ 33
\end{aligned}
$$

Total heat units: 189,337.5

This number of heat units is considerably more than the total capacity for this anode. Is it possible to use a comparable technique and allow for the safety factor of this anode? Change to a longer scale technique (you are going to exceed the 85 kVp rule for good contrast when using iodine as a contrast medium) and maybe it can be accomplished.

25 mAs
98 kVp } Equal technique, longer scale of contrast

Three-phase rectification

$$25 \times 98 \times 1.35 = 3307.5 \text{ HU per exposure}$$

$$(5737.5 - 3307.5 = 2430 \text{ HU savings per exposure})$$

$$3307.5 \times 33 = 109,147.5 \text{ total HU}$$

This program can be put safely on this anode with about 30,000 HU to spare.

How long must you wait after applying this program for this anode to cool? Notice the time in minutes on the bottom of the chart. Follow up the chart to about 110,000 HU. Move your finger over to the cooling line and notice about 1 minute left toward the left. Subtract that 1 minute from the total of 10 minutes and you determine that this anode cools in about 9 minutes. By following the cooling curve of this chart, you can see that the anode is capable of dissipating more heat faster when it is close to full capacity. (Notice that the cooling curve is more curved at the upper portion and assumes a straighter line further down.) It takes about 5 minutes to cool down from 50,000 HU and only 10 minutes to cool down from 140,000 HU. If this tube was heated to 90,000 HU, how long would it take to cool to just under 10,000 HU? Find the 90,000 HU on the left of the chart, follow it to the cooling curve, and record the time factor (2 minutes). Follow the curve to the 10,000-HU level; again, record the time (8-3/4 minutes). Subtract 2 minutes from 8-3/4 minutes; this tube will cool from 90,000 to 10,000 HU in 6-3/4 minutes. Now look at the cooling curve and begin at 140,000 HU. Follow the curve to 60,000 HU; it takes about 4 minutes to cool down to 60,000 HU. Both of these totals of dissipated heat units are 80,000, but it takes a shorter period of time to reduce the heat units by 80,000 when maximal heat is applied to the tube.

TUBE HOUSING COOLING

This type of chart demonstrates the number of heat units that can be stored within the x-ray tube housing. This housing is the structure that surrounds the actual tube. It consists of the outside covering of metal and a layer of lead, to protect the patient and the operator from excess x-radiation. Next, oil is used for insulation purposes. One of an operator's main concerns is to keep the oil below the boiling point. If the oil reaches this point, structural damage to the housing may occur and it could actually explode. This is usually not a problem with normal diagnostic radiography, but may become one when dealing with angiography, tomography, and cineradiography.

Notice Figure 15–4 and note that the heat units are higher for the tube housing cooling charts than for the anode thermal cooling charts. Notice that the time of cooling can be reduced by one half if an air circulator is used. This fan is located inside the tube housing and is activated whenever the heat in the housing reaches a certain temperature. You will know if the tube you are operating is equipped with a fan because you can hear it after the tube has been in use for some time.

Other tubes are cooled by removing the oil and replacing that oil with coded oil. This task is accomplished by sending the insulating oil through a series of tubing that leads both away from and back to the tube housing.

You will learn about more radiographic charts in a more advanced physics

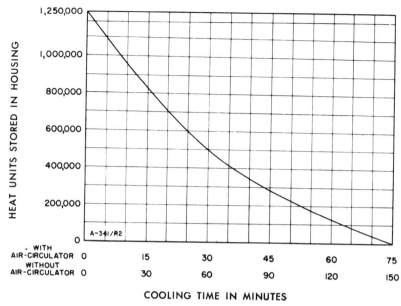

Fig. 15–4. Housing cooling chart. (Courtesy of Machlett Laboratories Inc., Springdale, CT.)

course. These charts are to be used when working with special radiographic procedures. These charts are used for *rapid film-sequence ratings* and mammography ratings.

As radiographers, by using tube rating and tube cooling charts correctly, you should be able to prolong the life of the x-ray tubes. These charts should be posted near the console of every radiography machine.

Radiographers can extend the life of x-ray tubes by one other means. Each tube should be warmed sufficiently before a heavy exposure is placed on the tube, especially when working with kVp ranges above 90. This procedure places a small amount of heat over the entire surface of the anode. Most x-ray tube manufacturers suggest a warm-up procedure for each tube in service. A good rule is to use about 65 to 75 kVp and a relatively long exposure time of somewhere between 1 and 2 seconds. Take three exposures with a delay time between each of about 30 seconds. These long exposure times allow the entire focal tract to be subjected to some portion of the exposure. These procedures are especially helpful when preserving a tube that is to be used with 100 kVp fluoroscopy or a 110-kVp chest radiograph. A considerable difference of opinion exists as to whether tubes that are utilized at 70- to 80-kVp range need to be warmed before using. Some authorities believe that by warming the anode you are only adding to the total heat units. I think that all radiographic tubes should be warmed for about 4 hours or more.

Radiographic tubes should be treated with care whenever they are used. Never move the tube quickly across the table and then stop it suddenly. These tubes should not be slammed or twisted from a vertical to a horizontal position, especially when the tube is hot. Such actions can cause separation of the filament. Once a filament has separated, it has lost contact and will no longer function. An x-ray tube can operate with only one filament, but it then operates with only one focal spot size.

1. List the three types of charts used in conjunction with radiographic tubes.

   Figure the heat units for the following:

2. 400 mA
   0.05 s
   98 kVp
   Single-phase
     equipment
   40-inch FFD

3. 600 mA
   40 ms
   90 kVp
   Three-phase
     equipment
   72-inch FFD

4. 20 mAs
   86 kVp
   Three-phase equipment
   4 Films per 5 seconds
   3 Films per 2 seconds
   2 Films per 4 seconds

5. How could you reduce the heat units to a tube without changing radiographic film density?

6. Why is tungsten used in the construction of radiographic tube anodes?

7. Rhenium is used in the construction of radiographic anodes because:
   1. It has a high melting point
   2. It keeps the anode from pitting
   3. It keeps the cathode from pitting
   a. All of the above   b. 1 Only   c. 2 Only   d. 1 and 3 Only

8. High-speed rotating anodes rotate at about _____ rpm.

9. Why is it usually not possible to overload a tube with one giant exposure?

10. Why should you strive to keep the x-ray exposures below the maximum allowed?

11. The anode is capable of dissipating more heat in a shorter time span:
    a. When it is heated to about one-half capacity
    b. When it is heated to capacity
    c. When it is heated to above capacity

12. The time of cooling for tube housings can be reduced by the use of _____.

13. What is the purpose of using a warm-up procedure for a radiographic tube?

14. An x-ray tube that is operating on only one filament has only one _____ _____ _____ that can be employed.

1. Application, Construction, Characteristics, and Care of X-Ray Screens. United States Radium Corporation, Brooklyn, NY 11218.
2. Bushong, S: *Radiologic Science for Technologists.* 4th ed. St. Louis, C.V. Mosby Co., 1988.
3. Characteristics and Applications of X-Ray Grids. Liebel-Flarsheim Co., 111 E. Amity Road, Cincinnati, OH 45215, 1968.
4. Cullinan, J: *Illustrated Guide to X-Ray Technics.* 2nd ed. Philadelphia, Lippincott, 1972.
5. Curry, TS, Dowdey, JE, Murry, RC: *Christensen's Introduction to the Physics of Diagnostic Radiology.* 3rd ed. Philadelphia, Lea & Febiger, 1984.
6. Fodor, J, Malott, J: *The Art and Science of Medical Radiography.* 6th ed. St. Louis, The Catholic Health Association of the United States, 1987.
7. Hiss, S: *Understanding Radiography.* Springfield, IL, Charles C Thomas, 1978.
8. How to Prepare an X-Ray Technic Chart. General Electric, Medical Systems Group, Box 414, Milwaukee, WI 53201.
9. How to Get Maximum Life from your Rotating Anode X-Ray Tubes. Machlett Laboratories, 1063 Hope Street, Springdale, CT 06907.
10. Selman, J: *The Fundamentals of X-Ray and Radium Physics.* 7th ed. Springfield, IL, Charles C Thomas, 1985.
11. Thompson, T: *Cahoon's Formulating X-Ray Techniques.* 9th ed. Durham, Duke University Press, 1979.
12. T-Grain Emulsion Advantage; Resolution without Compromise. Kodak Health Sciences, Rochester, NY, 1987.

Chapter 1

1. Electromagnetic
2. b. Short
3. Angstrom
4. 0.1, 0.5
5. Penetrating
6. Heat
7. Source or stream of electrons, set electron stream into motion, stop this electron stream very suddenly
8. Vacuum glass envelope, cathode, anode
9. Bone, liquid tissue, adipose tissue, and air tissue
10. Sufficient density, proper contrast, maximum detail, and minimum distortion

Chapter 2

1. mA, time, kVp, focal-film distance (FFD)
2. Milliamperage
3. 0.001 s (1 ms), 8 seconds
4. Seconds or milliseconds
5. 1000
6. Inversely
7. a. 15 b. 8 c. 5
8. a. 0.15 s 150 ms b. 0.05 s 50 ms c. 0.0083 s 8 ms
9. a. 1800 b. 400 c. 120
10. 1000
11. b. Shorter
12. d. 2 and 4
13. 2 × cm + 25 or 30; 25 for three-phase equipment; 30 for single-phase equipment
14. Lower than minimal kVp will not penetrate the object. Higher than normal tends to increase the scale of contrast.
15. Weaker

Chapter 3

1. Difference between the extreme blacks and whites of a radiographic image
2. Many subtle shades of gray on the radiograph
3. The image is mostly black and/or white
4. Long scale higher kVp produces more scattered and secondary radiation
5. a. High kVp—low mAs
6. a. 10 mAs, 101 kVp
   b. 0.0125 s, 89 kVp
   c. 18 ms, 92 kVp
   d. 200 mA, 103 kVp
7. a. 40 mAs, 75 kVp
   b. 0.006 s, 80 kVp
   c. 50 ms, 67 kVp
   d. 1600 mA, 68 kVp

Chapter 4

1. b. 2 and 3
2. $\dfrac{\text{Intensity 1} = \text{Distance 2}^2}{\text{Intensity 2} = \text{Distance 1}^2}$
3. $\dfrac{\text{Old mAs} = \text{Old FFD}^2}{\text{New mAs} = \text{New FFD}^2}$
4. 4.57 mrad
5. a. 31.6
   b. 0.05 s
   c. 0.03 s
   d. 36 ms
   e. 9 ms
6. 76 kVp, 4.88 mAs
7. 84 kVp, 94 ms
8. c. 600 mA, 1/60 s, 92 kVp
9. c. 200 mA, 1/10 s, 75 kVp

Chapter 5

1. We radiograph three-dimensional objects and place them as a two-dimensional image.
2. Geometric unsharpness, motion, material or inherent unsharpness, and magnification (size) unsharpness
3. c. Use a fast time
4. d. 400 mA, 0.05 s, 69 kVp
5. Most, b; least, c
6. Material or inherent
7. Because of divergence of light beam caused by the screens fluorescence
8. c. Thick films—angled central ray
9. a. 4.7 b. 6.35
10. a. 1.17 b. 1.05
11. a. 17.6% b. 5.8%
12. The image will be 10 × 12.5 inches. It will fit if it is angled on the film.
13. Shape distortion will move anatomic superimposition, allowing the radiologist to see anatomy free of this superimposition

Chapter 6

1. b. Heterogenous
2. c. Patient skin
3. b. 1, 2, and 3 only
4. Inherent and added or external filters
5. 2.5 mm aluminum equivalent
6. To equalize the patient density on the radiographic film
7. a. Cathode
8. b. Short
9. c. 11° angle of anode face
10. Use screen with different speeds in one cassette. The more dense tissue should be placed to coincide with the faster screen.
11. A wedge filter absorbs more x-radiation on the thicker side and gradually absorbs less toward the thin side. The trough allows more x-radiation to pass through the center of the filter and less through the lateral sides.
12. c. Posteroanterior projection of chest

Chapter 7

1. Gustave Bucky
2. b. Detail
3. a. The film
4. c. 12
5. Linear or parallel, focused, cross-hatch or criss-cross
6. Focused
7. The lines per inch or centimeter
8. d. High kVp techniques
9. Grid ratio =
$\dfrac{h}{D}$ height of lead strip
distance between lead strips
10. The one with 110 lines per inch
11. a. Increases
12. 6 mAs
13. a. 0.075 s b. 160 c. 101 mAs, so use 100

Chapter 8

1. Thomas Edison
2. b. Light produced by fluorescence
3. True. The image remains for a time after the exposure switch is released
4. Protective, active or phosphor, reflective, base
5. a. Faster. It helps to focus the light toward the film.

6. Fluorescent light
7. The intensifying screen will match the color spectrum of the film. The screen should fluoresce to whatever color the film is most sensitive.

8. Size and thickness
9. Speed
10. a. 26.4 b. 24
11. 29.4, so use 30
12. Screen films have less detail
13. a. 5 mAs b. 15 c. 0.125

Chapter 9

1. Protective, emulsion, adhesive, base, adhesive, emulsion, protective
2. Base
3. Larger crystals are faster than smaller size of the same composition
4. b. Less detail
5. d. 2 and 3
6. Patient dose of x-radiation
7. How much room for error with radiographic techniques
8. To produce gray films so the radiologist can see any small difference in tissue density
9. a. Breast

10. Roll film for spot radiography, video film, dental film, panoramic film, duplicating film, subtraction film, 16- or 35-mm cine film
11. Used for images produced by cathode ray tubes (computed tomography, ultrasonography, magnetic resonance imaging)
12. It is stronger and is not combustible
13. b. 1 only
14. True
15. c. Fog
16. c. 40–60%

Chapter 10

1. Cover up detail, increase density, increase patient dose of x-radiation, increase radiographer dose of x-radiation, make radiographs harder to interpret
2. d. 4
3. b. Behind
4. c. 3 only
5. d. 1 and 2
6. No
7. a. 3.6 × 3.6 inches b. 2.52 × 3.11

inches
8. The lead absorbs scattered and secondary radiation that would otherwise hit the film when the patient is in the lateral position. When the patient is supine the scattered and secondary radiation is absorbed by the patient.
9. Use 50% more mAs than for the 14 × 17-inch film

Chapter 11

1. d. Caucasian women
2. a. More
3. a. A higher
4. b. Lower. Because of the scattered and secondary radiation produced in the water tissue of children.

5. 12 years
6. a. 8.75 mAs, 58 kVp or 4.37 mAs, 67 kVp
   b. 14 mAs, 54 kVp or 7 mAs, 62 kVp
   c. 300 mA, 73 kVp or 150 mA, 84 kVp

7. a. 12 mAs, 55 kVp or 6 mAs, 63
       kVp
    b. 5 mAs, 64 kVp or 2.5 mAs, 74
       kVp
    c. 0.028 s, 84 kVp or 0.014 s, 97
       kVp
8. So you can use a short exposure
    time
9. Grandmother. This person only
    receives somatic x-radiation. Even
    staff radiographers past child-
    bearing age should not be used
    because radiographers work in an
    x-radiation environment.
10. b. Poor, weak
11. 25–30%
12. 15.4 to 16.5 or use one half this
    mAs and add 15% to the kVp.
13. The shoulder can vary greatly
    from patient to patient. There-
    fore, exercise care when radi-
    ographing this area. It is a good
    idea to always check the first x-
    ray exposure for proper tech-
    nique.

Chapter 12

1. So you have some idea of the pa-
    thology involved
2. b. Decrease
3. d. 30
4. a. 5
5. a. Increase. Because emphysema
    is caused by the addition of
    exudate or fluid within the pa-
    tient.
6. Wheezing type of breathing;
    barrel-shaped chest
7. About 83
8. About 17.5

Chapter 13

1. b. Density
2. False
3. a. It does not penetrate the anat-
    omy adequately
    b. It makes the radiograph too
    gray or flat looking
4. d. 800
5. Ionization chamber
6. c. 2 only
7. b. Insufficient density at the
    lumbar area
8. The air is most likely located just
    above the photo cell. Thus the
    cell received enough radiation
    to shut off the exposure before
    the other areas of the film re-
    ceived sufficient x-radiation for
    proper density.

Chapter 14

1. d. 3 only
2. a. 2 times
3. d. 85
4. a. Use 6 to 8 more kVp
5. Variable kVp; fixed kVp
6. 2 × cm + 25 for three-phase
    equipment; 2 × cm + 30 for sin-
    gle-phase equipment
7. b. 2
8. b. 20% more mAs
9. Fixed kVp
10. They produce a longer scale of
    contrast, which is good for chest
    radiography. The radiologist is
    able to see smaller tissue den-
    sity differences in the radio-
    graph.

Chapter 15

1. Tube rating chart, anode cooling chart, tube housing cooling chart
2. 1960
3. 2916
4. 78,948
5. Use higher kVp 15% and reduce the mAs by one half
6. Because of its high melting point and its high atomic number
7. c. 2 only
8. 10,000
9. Because of circuit breakers
10. To prolong the life of the x-ray tube
11. When heated to capacity. It should never be heated above capacity.
12. Air circulating fans or oil that can be removed and returned to the tube housing
13. So the anode surface is operating at equal temperatures, which should prolong the life of the tube
14. Focal spot size

GENERAL REVIEW QUESTIONS

1. X-rays penetrate all matter according to its _____.

2. List eight properties of x-rays.

3. The quality of an x-ray beam depends on the _____.
   1. mA   2. Time   3. kVp   4. FFD
   a. 1 and 2   b. 3 and 4   c. 3 only   d. 1, 2, and 3
                  e. All of the above

4. The quantity of an x-ray beam depends on the _____.
   1. mA   2. Time   3. kVp   4. FFD
   a. 1 and 2   b. 3 and 4   c. 1 only   d. 3 only
                  e. All of the above

5. mA is _____ proportional to the exposure time:
   a. Directly   c. Inversely
   b. Indirectly   d. Approximately

6. Radiographs of the chest or stomach should use an exposure time of:
   a. Less than 1 second   c. 1/10 second or more
   b. Less than 1/10 second   d. 1/10 second or less

7. Long scale contrast films demonstrate:
   a. Black and white shades   c. More black than white shades
   b. Gray shades   d. More white than black shades

8. Short scale contrast films demonstrate:
   a. Black and white shades   c. More white than black shades
   b. More white than black shades d. Gray shades

9. _____ scale contrast is usually more beneficial to the patient.
   a. Long   b. Short   c. Any

10. a. State the rule of thumb for determining minimum kVp.
    b. Why do most departments use more kVp than this?

11. In order to maintain equal film density, if the distance is doubled, the mAs must be _____.
    a. × 2   b. × 4   c. ÷ 2   d. ÷ 4

12. Which film image demonstrates the best detail?
    a. Supine chest 40-inch FFD   c. Lateral lumbar spine
    b. Erect chest 72-inch FFD   d. Fluoro spots

13. No amount of mAs can compensate for insufficient _____.

14. An inherent filter is composed of what?

15. X-rays are composed of _____ wavelengths.
    a. Heterogenous   b. Homogenous

16. Radiographic filters render the wavelengths _____.
    a. Softer   b. Harder   c. Longer   d. Wider   e. Easier to be absorbed

17. Which of the following would benefit the **most** from a compensating filter?
    a. Hand   b. Normal chest   c. Knee   d. Foot

18. A _____ x-ray beam is more penetrating.
    a. Long wavelength   b. Short wavelength

19. A _____ x-ray beam will be more absorbed by the skin.
    a. Hardened   b. Softened

20. The _____ the kVp, the longer the wavelengths of the x-ray photons.
    a. Higher   b. Lower

21. An external filter has the most beneficial effect on the _____.
    a. Internal organs   c. Gonads
    b. Blood cells   d. Skin

22. Explain how heel effect can benefit your technique for a thoracic spine image:
    a. In the anteroposterior position.
    b. In the lateral position.

23. If different screens are used for compensating filters, how would you use one on a patient with pneumonia on the left side?

24. Where on the radiographic machine would you place a wedge compensating filter for radiography?

25. Geometric unsharpness depends on:
    a. FFD, focal spot size, object-film distance (OFD)
    b. FFD, intensifying screens, OFD
    c. Focal spot size, FFD, intensifying screens
    d. Focal spot size, OFD, intensifying screens
    e. Focal spot size, FOD, intensifying screens

26. What are the three types of radiographic unsharpness?

27. Which is the worst of the types of unsharpness listed in question 26?

28. Anterior ribs demonstrate more geometric unsharpness radiographed with the patient in the _____ position.
    a. Prone
    b. Supine

29. By using a long FFD, the geometric unsharpness is:
    a. More
    b. Less
    c. The same

30. The object-film distance (OFD) should be as short as possible when taking radiographs.
    ( ) True
    ( ) False

31. A _____ FFD is beneficial to the x-ray tube.
    a. Long
    b. Short

32. Which technique is more beneficial to the **patient?**
    a. 100 kVp,   60 mAs, 40-inch FFD
    b. 90 kVp, 120 mAs, 40-inch FFD
    c. 110 kVp,   30 mAs, 40-inch FFD

33. The _____ of the x-ray beam increases as the FFD increases.
    a. Intensity
    b. Width
    c. Visibility
    d. Penetration
    e. Wavelengths

34. Grids reduce scattered and secondary radiation from reaching what?

35. What is meant by grid ratio?

36. A focused grid with a focus range of 31 to 37 inches produces the best radiographic images at _____ inches.

37. Grid cut-off is apparent when the tube is angled how?

38. Parallax effect is more visible on which type of films:
    a. Long FFD, angled central ray
    b. Short FFD, angled central ray
    c. Short FFD, 1 central ray
    d. Long FFD, 1 central ray

39. Which film will have the shortest scale contrast:
    a. 200 mAs, 16:1 grid
    b. 100 mAs, 6:1 grid
    c. 120 mAs, 8:1 grid

40. List the layers of an intensifying screen.

41. Screen type film is more sensitive to the action of:
    1. Yellow light   2. X-rays   3. Blue-violet light   4. Green light
    a. All the above   b. 2 only   c. 2, 3, 4   d. 3 and 4   e. 3 only

42. When using intensifying screens about _____% of the image is produced by x-rays.
    a. 5   b. 20   c. 30   d. 40   e. 95

43. The _____ layer of an intensifying screen is the same as the phosphor layer.
    a. Reflective   b. Active   c. Shining   d. Abrasion

44. The _____ the active layer of an intensifying screen, the slower the screen.
    a. Thicker   b. Thinner

45. High-speed intensifying screens require:
    a. Less radiation than medium speed for the same results
    b. Less radiation than slow speed for the same results
    c. More radiation than medium speed but less than detail for the same results
    d. All the above
    e. a and b but not c

46. Fast screens have a limitation of _____.
    a. The image   c. Fluorescence
    b. Detail   d. Crystal

47. Penumbra is the:
    a. True image   c. Sharpness of a radiograph
    b. False image   d. Blurriness of the film edges

48. When is the latent image present on a radiograph film?

49. Why is a collimator better than a cone for reducing scattered and secondary radiation?

50. How much technique change is needed to change from a field size of 14 × 17 to a 10 × 12-inch field size?

The following technique was used for an abdomen film:

100 mA, 3/10 s, 84 kVp. The patient measurement is 21 cm.

51. What technique should you use for a child of 2 months with a measurement of 7 cm? (abdomen)

52. For a 3-year-old child with a measurement of 14 cm? (abdomen)

53. For a 9-year-old child with a measurement of 17 cm? (abdomen)

54. For a 14 × 17-inch, anteroposterior film of barium-filled bowel in a patient with a 21-cm measurement?

55. For an anteroposterior projection of the lumbar spine if the measurement is 20 cm?

56. For a post-fatty meal gallbladder, if the measurement is 24 cm?
    The following are diseases that necessitate the use of different than normal radiographic techniques. What are the corrective factors that should be used?

57. Arthritis:

58. Paget's disease:

59. Emphysema:

60. Atrophy:

61. Osteoporosis:
    Solve for the unknown:

62. 660 mA, 50 ms, mAs = ?

63. 500 mA, 0.06 s, mAs = ?

64. 25 mAs, 1/50 s, mA = ?

65. 30 mAs, 0.03 s, mA = ?

66. 40 mAs, 800 mA, s = ?

67. 5 mAs, 300 mA, ms = ?

68. A long scale film = 80 kVp, 60 mAs. Shorten the scale of contrast and use 1/10 s time: kVp = ?   mA = ?

69. A short scale film = 76 kVp, 40 mAs. Lengthen the scale of contrast and use 200 mA: kVp = ?   s = ?

Keep density equal in the following:

Old Technique	New Technique
70. 40-inch FFD 100 mAs	60-inch FFD ? mAs 500 mA ? s
71. 72-inch FFD 50 mAs 1/10 s	40-inch FFD ? mAs 1/20 s ? mA
72. 50-inch FFD 50 mAs 100 film/screen combination 8:1 grid	44-inch FFD ? mAs 400 film/screen combination 12:1 grid

Figure the geometric unsharpness for the following:

73. FSS = 2   74. FSS = 0.5   75. FSS = 0.3
    OFD = 10   OFD = 4   OFD = 10
    FFD = 40   FOD = 36   FFD = 72

Figure the magnification for the following:

76. Object size: 6 × 8   77. Object size: 5
    FFD = 40   FFD = 36
    OFD = 6   FOD = 31
    Image = ?   % magnification = ?

78. What is the magnification factor for the following:
    44-inch FFD, 6-inch OFD?

79. Which technique is equal to 1/10 s, 100 mA, 50 kVp, no grid:
    a. 2/10 s, 50 mA, 50 kVp, 5:1 grid
    b. 2/10 s, 100 mA, 58 kVp, 12:1 grid

c. 2/10 s, 200 mA, 50 kVp, 8:1 grid
d. None of the above

80. Which technique equals the most density?
    a. 100 mAs, 60 kVp, no grid
    b. 500 mAs, 60 kVp, 12:1 grid
    c. 400 mAs, 60 kVp, 8:1 grid
    d. 100 mAs, 68 kVp, 5:1 grid
    e. 300 mAs, 72 kVp, 6:1 grid

81. Which technique equals the least density?
    a. 100 mA, 1/2 s, 80 kVp, 16:1 grid
    b. 200 mA, 1/2 s, 80 kVp, 8:1 grid
    c. 300 mA, 1/10 s, 82 kVp, 16:1 grid
    d. 400 mA, 1/20 s, 90 kVp, 12:1 grid

82. What is the intensifying factor for the following intensifying screen?
    Exposure with screens = 20 mAs
    Exposure without screens = 260 mAs

Figure the field size for the following:

83. 40-inch FFD
    6-inch diameter of cone
    16-inch distance from target to
        bottom of cone

84. 72-inch FFD
    1 × 2.5 cone size
    12-inch distance from target to
        bottom of cone

Figure the diaphragm size for the following:

85. Field size = 9 × 9
    FFD = 40
    Target to diaphragm = 14

86. Field size = 8 × 10
    FFD = 30
    Target to diaphragm = 12

87. 30 mAs at 77 kVp is a good technique for an abdomen film on a patient with a measurement of 23 cm. What should you use for a lumbar spine film (anteroposterior projection)?

88. For an intravenous pyelogram, 10-minute film on the same patient (14 × 17-inch field size).

89. For a barium enema, right anterior oblique, on the same patient (14 × 17-inch field size).

90. The overall blackening of a radiograph is called _____.

91. The highest kVp that should be used with iodine as a contrast medium is _____.

92. Why should you be concerned with kVp if you are using a machine with phototiming?

93. Calcifications in the urinary tract are:
    1. Radiopaque   2. Radiolucent   3. Visible on the scout film
              4. Visible on the contrast film
    a. 1 and 2   c. 1, 2, and 4
    b. 1, 2, and 3   d. 1 only
                        e. All the above

94. A patient receives 24 mrad at a point 40 inches from a source. If you stand 8 feet from this same source, how many millirad would you receive?

95. What is the best way to combat motion caused by peristalsis?

96. A cervical spine radiograph (anteroposterior view) is taken with the following factors:
40-inch FFD, 12 mAs, 68 kVp, 12:1 grid
What technique would you use for a 72-inch lateral with a 6:1 grid?

97. What could cause material unsharpness?
1. Films   2. Screen   3. Motion   4. Object-film distance
a. All the above   c. 3 only
b. 1 only   d. 1 and 2
              e. 1, 2, and 3

98. List the four tissue types found in the body. Start with the least radiopaque.

99. X-ray beams are measured in _____ units.

100. List the four basic qualities that should be demonstrated on all radiographic images.

101. What is the rule of thumb to determine minimum kVp?

102. What is the grid ratio for the following:
Height of lead strip = 0.25 mm
Space between lead strip = 0.025

103. Why are low ratio grids used in conjunction with fluoroscopy but higher ratio grids are usually used for the overhead projections?

104. Explain the term luminescence.

105. An 800 film/screen combination produces a film with a _____ scale of contrast than a 400 film/screen combination.
a. Shorter   b. Longer

106. Poor screen contact resembles _____ on the radiographic image.
a. Motion   c. Long scale contrast
b. Magnification   d. Short scale contrast

107. The two most important film characteristics for the radiographer are _____ and _____.

108. Very long scale contrast films are excellent for examination of which of the following:
a. Gastrointestinal tract   c. Chests
b. Extremities   d. Skull

109. Another name for crossover radiation is _____.

110. The proper name for duplication film is _____.

111. List two distinct advantages of polyester over cellulose acetate as a radiographic film base.

112. The main disadvantage to using nonscreen film is _____.

113. A modern collimator usually works with _____ main lead shutters.
    a. 2   b. 4   c. 6   d. 8

114. A _____% of increase or decrease in mAs makes a visible difference on the radiographic image.
    a. 5   b. 15   c. 20   d. 30

115. A _____% increase or decrease in kVp makes a visible difference in the radiographic density.
    a. 5   b. 10   c. 15   d. 20   e. 25

116. The most accurate type of automatic exposure control device is the _____.

117. When working with a fixed kVp radiographic technique chart, a _____% increase in mAs is used when going from medium-sized patients to large patients.
    a. 10   b. 20   c. 30   d. 40

118. The normal centimeter measurement for an adult lateral skull is about _____.

119. Low-speed rotating anodes usually rotate at about _____ rpm.
    a. 2600   b. 3600   c. 10,000   d. 20,000

Figure the heat units for the following:

120. 500 mA	121. 800 mA	122. 10 mAs
50 ms	1/50 s	80 kVp
80 kVp	92 kVp	Three-phase
Three-phase	Single-phase	equipment
equipment	equipment	3 films per second/
40-inch FFD	36-inch FFD	3 seconds
		2 films per second/
		3 seconds
		1 film per second/
		4 seconds

123. How can heat units be reduced without altering the density?

124. The time of cooling for the tube housing can be reduced by the use of:
    1. Circulating fans   2. Removing and replacing insulating oil
    3. Increasing the anode rotating speed
    a. 1 only   b. 1 and 2 only   c. 1 and 3 only   d. All the above

125. Which film will produce the most radiographic density?
  a. 60 mAs
     85 kVp
     40-inch FFD
     8:1 grid
     800 film/screen combination

  b. 800 mA
     0.1 s
     80 kVp
     50-inch FFD
     6:1 grid
     400 film/screen combination

  c. 600 mA
     1/30 s
     92 kVp
     45-inch FFD
     12:1 grid
     200 film/screen combination

ANSWER KEY TO GENERAL REVIEW QUESTIONS

1. Density
2. List from page (1–3)
3. c. 3 only
4. a. 1 and 2
5. c. Inversely
6. b. Less than 1/10 second
7. b. Gray shades
8. a. Black and white shades
9. a. Long
10. a. 2 × cm + 25 or 30
    b. To get a longer scale of contrast or so the patient receives less x-radiation
11. b. × 4
12. b. Erect chest 72-inch FFD
13. kVp
14. Oil, glass, collimator mirrors
15. a. Heterogenous
16. b. Harder
17. d. Foot
18. b. Short wavelength
19. b. Softened
20. b. Lower
21. d. Skin
22. a. Place anode above upper or less dense area of thoracic spine
    b. Place anode above lower or less dense area of thoracic spine
23. Place the pneumonia side (left)

so it coincides with the higher speed screen
24. Under the collimator
25. a. FFD, focal spot size, OFD
26. Motion, inherent, geometric
27. Motion
28. b. Supine
29. b. Less
30. True
31. b. Short
32. c. 110 kVp, 30 mAs, 40-inch FFD
33. b. Width
34. The film
35. Grid ratio is height over distance. $GR = \dfrac{h}{D}$
36. 34
37. Across the lead strips
38. b. Short FFD, angled central ray
39. a. 200 mAs, 16:1 grid
40. Abrasion-active or phosphor-reflective-base or backing
41. d. 3 and 4
42. a. 5
43. b. Active
44. b. Thinner
45. e. a and b but not c
46. b. Detail
47. d. Blurriness of the film edges
48. After exposure, before develop-

ing
49. Because it removes the off-focus or stem radiation
50. 20% more mAs
51. 4.5 mAs, 64 kVp or 2.25 mAs, 74 kVp
52. 18 mAs, 70 kVp or 9 mAs, 80 kVp or 4.5 mAs, 92 kVp
53. 27 mAs, 76 kVp or 13.5 mAs, 86 kVp
54. 30 mAs, 93 kVp or 15 mAs, 107 kVp
55. 36 mAs, 82 kVp
56. 80 mAs, 76 kVp
57. Down about 6 to 8 kVp
58. Up about 6 to 8 kVp
59. Down about 6 to 10 kVp
60. Down about 6 to 8 kVp
61. Down about 6 to 8 kVp
62. 33
63. 30
64. 1250
65. 1000
66. 0.05
67. 16.6 or 17
68. 68 kVp, 1200 mA
69. 87 kVp, 0.1 s
70. 225 mAs, 0.45 s
71. 15.4 mAs, 308 mA
72. 12.1 mAs
73. 2/3 or 0.66
74. 1/18 or 0.055
75. 3/62 or 0.0483
76. 7 × 9.4
77. 16
78. 1.15
79. c. 2/10 s, 200 mA, 50 kVp, 8:1 grid
80. e. 300 mAs, 72 kVp, 6:1 grid
81. c. 300 mA, 1/10 s, 82 kVp, 16:1 grid
82. 13
83. 15
84. 6 × 15
85. 3.15 × 3.15
86. 4 × 3.2
87. 36 mAs, 77 kVp
88. 30 mAs, 80 kVp or 6 mAs, 70 kVp
89. 30 mAs, 93 kVp or 15 mAs, 107 kVp

90. Density
91. 85
92. You must have sufficient kVp to penetrate the object and not too much so the image will be too gray
93. c. 1, 2, and 4
94. 4.1
95. Use a high mA station so a short exposure time can be used
96. 2.2 mAs, 68 kVp
97. d. 1 and 2
98. Air, fat or adipose, liquid, bone
99. Ångstrom
100. Proper contrast, sufficient density, maximum detail, minimal distortion
101. 2 × cm measurement + 25 or 30
102. 10:1
103. Because the area radiographed is small, so less scattered and secondary radiation is produced
104. To glow with stimulation
105. a. Shorter
106. a. Motion
107. Latitude and speed
108. c. Chest
109. Punch-through
110. Solarization
111. Strength, noncombustible
112. Radiation dose to the patient
113. b. 4
114. d. 30
115. a. 5
116. Ionization chamber
117. c. 30
118. 14
119. b. 3600
120. 2700
121. 1472
122. 20,520
123. Use a longer scale of contrast
124. b. 1 and 2 only
125. b. 800 mA, 0.1 s, 80 kVp, 50-inch FFD, 6:1 grid, 400 film/screen combination.

Index

Page numbers in italics indicate figures.

Photo cell(s), 103–105, *104*
Polyester
    as film base, 70
Punch-through radiation, 72

Radiation
    crossover (punch-through), 72
    scattered
        effects of, 46
    secondary
        effects of, 46
    stem (off-focus), 77
Radiographic contrast. *See* Contrast
Radiographic exposure. *See* Exposure
Radiographic film. *See* Film(s)
Radiographic filter(s). *See* Filter(s)
Radiographic grid(s). *See* Grid(s)
Radiographic technique chart(s), 108–120,
    113–114
    fixed kVp, 116–117
    high kVp, 116
    variable kVp, 109–116, *110–112*
Radiographic unsharpness. *See* Unsharpness
Radiography
    geriatric, 89–91
    orthopedic cast, 99–100
    pediatric, 91–94
Rare earth screen(s), 60, 61
Restraint(s)
    for children, *92–93,* 92–94
    for elderly patients, 90
Rhenium
    in anode construction, 122
Roll film, 71

Scattered radiation
    effects of, 46
Shape distortion, 31–32, *32*
Skull
    variable kVp technique chart
        preparation for, 114–115
Solarization film, 72
Spectral matching, 60

Static, *72,* 73
Stem radiation, 77
Subtraction film, 72

Time of exposure, 8–10
    back-up
        with automatic exposure control device, 103
Tissue(s)
    density of different types of, 2, *3*
Trough filter(s), 42
Tungsten
    in anode construction, 122

Unsharpness, 26–35
    geometric, 27–29
    inherent, 29–30
    magnification, 30–31
    motion, 26–27
    shape, 31–32, *32*
    types of, 26

Video film, 71

Wedge filter(s), 41, *41*
Wire mesh test
    for film screen contact, 65, *65*

X-ray(s), 1
    divergence of, 11, 20, *21*
    hardened, 36
    production of, 1–2, *2*
    properties of, 2–4
    purposes of medical use of, 2
    useful range of, 1
X-ray tube(s), 1–2, *2*
    care of, 121–128
    cost of, 121
    filaments of, *28,* 122–123
    housing cooling charts for, 126, *127*
    means for extending life of, 127
    rating charts for, 123–124, *123–124*
    thermal capacity of, 122
    warm–up procedure for, 127